Lighten up

Lighten up

365 Ways to Lose Weight and Feel Great

ANDREW CATE

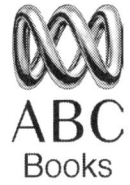

ABC
Books

Published by ABC Books for the
AUSTRALIAN BROADCASTING CORPORATION
GPO BOX 9994 Sydney NSW 2001

First published January 2008

National Library of Australia
Cataloguing in Publication entry
Cate, Andrew.
    Lighten up : 365 ways to lose fat fast.
    ISBN 9780733322525 (pbk.).
    1. Diet - Health aspects. 2. Exercise - Health aspects. 3. Weight loss - Health aspects.
    4. Health - Nutritional aspects. I. Australian Broadcasting Authority. II. Title.
    613.2

Cover and internal design by Wendy Farley, Anthouse
Typeset in 9pt on 11pt Helvetica Neue
Printed in Australia by Griffin Press, South Australia

5 4 3 2 1

Dedication

To my parents, for a lifetime of love and support.
Thank you always.

Introduction ... to a new approach

THIS BOOK is the culmination of more than 15 years of work as a personal trainer, weight-loss coach and health and fitness writer. It includes all the tips, tools and training techniques I know can help you lose weight and get results.

But more importantly, it gets you to look at weight loss from a totally different perspective. Isn't it worth putting a bit more time towards something that would dramatically improve the quality and quantity of your life? Isn't it worth more than just a few weeks on a crazy diet that you know you can't stick to?

Think about the tortoise and the hare. It's easy to be tempted to race off at 100 kilometres an hour and seek out fast results. But that approach is almost certain to fail. All it leaves you with is a few extra kilos a month or two down the track. A slow and steady approach is not so flashy, but it's much more likely to be successful. It won't happen overnight, but it will happen.

Inside *Lighten Up* you'll find 365 ways to help you lose weight, trim body fat and boost your energy levels. *Lighten Up* has been written to consistently and progressively inform, educate and motivate you in three key areas – attitude, food and movement. The book is focused on giving you proven facts on how to lose weight but also, and more importantly, giving you practical ways you can apply this knowledge to your life. That's why you'll find a 'Living it' section on every page of *Lighten Up*.

I encourage you to read *Lighten Up* like a tortoise, just one slow, steady step at a time. Think about each topic and how it applies to you. That way, you can absorb the information and live it progressively, instead of feeling overwhelmed. If that doesn't suit you, you could always read seven tips a day, and transform *Lighten Up* into an 8-week program. That's still a realistic amount of time to make some changes and kick-start your journey. Either way, try slowing down a little to get ahead. Enjoy the journey.

Andrew Cate

Day 1 tip – Motivation and mindset

Take one small step today. One giant leap for your health and body shape

Taking one small step is where every great journey begins. While you tend to hear a lot about where a journey starts and where it ends, it's the small steps along the way that get you there. You are about to embark on such a journey to a better body and better health, so congratulations on starting. This book is virtually guaranteed to help you lose weight; however, in order to complete that journey, turn your attention towards the steps you need to take along the way.

Living it

As you progress through *Lighten Up*, try to pick out at least one strategy or thinking habit that you will adopt each day or each week. Don't try to do too much too early because you will get better results by focusing on only one or two things at a time. One step leads you closer to the next step. Try to fight that little part of yourself that wants to know it all now, start like a bull at gate, and have results by yesterday. Haven't you tried that before without much success? So for today, and for the rest of your journey with *Lighten Up*, concentrate on mastering one thing at a time.

Day 2 tip – Good food

Make food the solution, not the problem

Whether you are concerned about losing fat, or just maximising your health and vitality, food is the key ingredient. Eating good food will increase your chances of getting great results. Healthier eating is not about perfection, or lettuce leaves. Healthy eating can still be enjoyable. As you become accustomed to it, healthy eating can be one of life's true pleasures.

Living it

Learn to get control over food instead of letting it control you. There are no good foods or bad foods, but there are some foods that I encourage you to eat more of and some to eat less of. Throughout this book you'll find loads of information on strategies to regain control over food, but try these to begin with:

- Plan your meals
- Shop to a list
- Freeze healthy meals so they are easily available

- Keep a food diary
- Aim for a lifetime eating plan, not a diet
- Involve your immediate family (the people you eat with regularly)
- Manage your stress, and find ways to relax
- Create a no-fail, no-willpower-required healthy environment at home
- Don't deprive yourself of anything, just use small portions of treats
- Start with small dietary changes and build week by week.

Day 3 tip – Move more

See your doctor before starting an exercise program (conditions apply)

You probably realise I am going to encourage you to start moving more. But there are some circumstances where you should consult your doctor for a medical examination before you start. You'll be glad to know that it's pretty rare that a doctor will encourage you not to exercise. In fact, it's been said that if you could bottle all the benefits of exercise, it would be the most heavily prescribed medication in the world.

Living it

See your doctor before you start to exercise if you:

- are aged 55 years or older
- have had a previous heart attack or stroke
- are very overweight
- are a heavy smoker
- have a medical condition such as diabetes, asthma, arthritis or high blood pressure
- are taking prescribed medication
- have a family history of heart disease
- are pregnant, or have given birth in the last 6 weeks
- have any doubts about your health.

Once you have clearance from your doctor, or even if you don't, begin gradually and ease your body back into regular activity.

Day 4 tip – Motivation and mindset

If you eat it, burn it. If you drink it, earn it

Get a grasp of this heading, and you'll go a long way towards getting a handle on the key ingredient to losing weight and fat. That ingredient is changing your energy balance (or kilojoule balance). Whatever kilojoules you eat or drink, you need to burn them off, and then a little extra. The problem I see regularly is that when people hear the words energy balance, or kilojoule balance, they switch off. No matter how important it is, there just doesn't seem to be any relevance. So to keep things practical, try to remember the heading of this tip. Burn off what you eat, and earn any extra kilojoules you drink with physical activity. Get this right, and your fat cells will have no choice but to get smaller.

Living it

If you burn off more kilojoules than you consume on at least 4 days out of every 7, more often than not you will be removing stored body fat. But try to be aware of your kilojoule balance on a daily basis, and make adjustments to your kilojoule intake and expenditure to keep it under control. Use the tips in this book to find ways to minimise your kilojoule intake (without starving yourself) and maximise the kilojoules you burn off each day.

Day 5 tip – Good food

Cut back on how many kilojoules you eat

People get fat by eating too many kilojoules, and not burning off enough. To reverse the process and lose fat, you need to consume less kilojoules and burn off more. You need to create a kilojoule deficit, so you burn off not just the kilojoules you eat, but also tap into the reserve of excess kilojoules stored as body fat. The key is to eat enough protein and fibre to fill you up and minimise hunger. Let's face it; the only way you will stick to dietary changes over the long-term is if you are always hungry.

Living it

It's simply not possible to lose body fat without cutting back on your kilojoule intake. What high-kilojoule components of your diet can you change or improve upon? Here are some changes that would help reduce your kilojoule intake (we'll talk more about them throughout the book):

- Fill out your meals with water-rich vegetables
- Add spice to your lunches and dinners
- Drink water before and during your meals

- Reduce your alcohol intake and have alcohol-free days
- Cut out fruit juice, or at least water it down
- Have low-carbohydrate dinners, or at least use low GI carbohydrates.

Day 6 tip – Move more

Move more than you do now

To genuinely remove existing stores of body fat and keep it off, you need to get physically active with both planned and incidental movement. Physical activity burns kilojoules, and burning kilojoules burns fat. Even light-intensity activities such as gardening, household cleaning and slow walking can burn kilojoules. I like to start off using the term 'movement' because it sounds less daunting than exercise. Move more, and you lose more.

Living it

As you read through *Lighten Up*, you'll learn about the best time of day to be active, the best type of activity, how often, and how hard you should push yourself. But for now, the most important thing is that you do something, start somewhere, and move your body more than you are moving it now. Walking is a great starting point because it's free, you can do it anywhere, and you already have all the equipment you need – legs. If you are already active, just increase what you are doing a little. Burn off more kilojoules this week than you did last week. We'll fine tune your exercise throughout the book.

Day 7 tip – Motivation and mindset

Start today and don't delay. The sooner you start, the better

When someone is overweight their body develops a memory for that specific level of body fat. This is often referred to as a 'settling or set point'. The longer the extra weight remains, the more comfortable the body becomes with it there, and the stronger your body will be at defending that 'set point' of fat. Because of this set point, anyone who has been overweight in the past will find it a little easier to regain body fat in the future. That is unless there are permanent lifestyle changes. So the sooner you lose weight, and the more permanent the changes that you make, the easier it will be.

Living it

While it's never too late to improve you health and body shape, the younger you start to lose body fat, the easier it will be to get results.

Day 8 tip – Good food

Go on a diet, as long as it's for life

Diets that promise fast weight loss may be popular, but they are rarely effective. Diets attract attention by offering miracle results, with gimmicky rules or restrictions that seem different, or 'too good to be true'. People usually go on a diet with the underlying intention of returning to their old habits as quickly as possible. People ditch their new diet because of boredom, deprivation, lack of energy, constipation or hunger. There are no laws that require a fad diet to be effective, factual or safe. One thing you can rely on is that the faster you lose weight, the faster it will return. That's part of the problem with fad diets – they are a fad. Short-term changes in your diet will only lead to short-term changes in your body shape.

Living it

There is no ideal way to eat, which is why there are so many different diets. The solution is to gradually find your own way, seeking to adapt, modify and experiment with food. Try to develop a way of eating that is easy to live with, forever. This is sometimes called a lifetime eating plan. The way you eat and exercise to lose weight has to be the way you live when you have lost weight. The best diet secret you will ever learn is that there is no magic diet.

Day 9 – Move more

Warm up before you exercise (it can help you burn more kilojoules)

The purpose of a warm-up is to prepare your body for exercise, and ease you from a resting state into an active one. The gradual increase in your heart rate helps to deliver more oxygen and glucose to your muscles, which can increase your level of performance during exercise, and burn more kilojoules. It can also help to prevent soft tissue injuries, which could interrupt the momentum of your exercise program.

Living it

A warm-up should focus on elevating your heart rate for around 5 minutes using the muscles that are part of your planned activity. If your activity is gentle, such as walking or cycling, just start at a slower speed for the first few minutes. If your activity is intense, and includes sprinting or very heavy lifting, it may be beneficial to do some stretches after you have elevated your heart rate. Never stretch cold. The importance of your warm-up also will depend on the air temperature. When it's cold, it takes longer to warm up your muscles, so increase the duration of your warm-up.

Day 10 tip – Motivation and mindset

Have a clear, positive, long-term goal to strive for

Setting goals is one of the most under-used strategies for weight control, but one of the most important. You can have the desire, but without a specific target to aim for you can easily miss the mark. Goal setting gives you direction and motivation, helping you to work systematically and progressively towards an end result.

Living it

Setting a long-term goal helps to focus your attention, linking knowledge and desire to purpose and action. Setting a goal to lose 10 kilos in 12 months is okay, but your focus is negative. To get over the hurdles and obstacles that will be part of every weight-loss journey, it helps to have a positive focus. I have listed some positive long-term goals below, but it's important to think long and hard about what will drive you. Your level of desire to achieve this goal will ultimately determine your level of success.

- Compete in a local fun run, and beat a set time.
- Compete in a marathon, triathlon, big swim or endurance paddling event.
- Walk or cycle between two distant towns, suburbs or beaches.
- Walk to Cradle Mountain in Tasmania.
- Complete the Kokoda Track in Papua New Guinea.
- Exercise 6 days a week for 12 weeks.
- Walk the Milford Sound in New Zealand.

Day 11 tip – Good food

Know your kilojoules from your calories

Kilojoules and calories measure the total energy value of foods. Australia uses kilojoules, but calories are still used as a measurement in the United States. One calorie is equivalent to 4.2 kilojoules. Our bodies need roughly 5500–6500 kilojoules per day, although this will vary depending on your age, weight, height and activity levels. It's estimated we need to eat at least 5000 kilojoules (1200 calories) to get enough nutrients in our diet and keep our metabolism functioning well. To burn off one kilogram of body fat in a week, you would need to create a kilojoule deficit of 38,000 kilojoules (9000 calories), or around 5500 kilojoules a day. That's why fat loss is a slow process.

Living it

I understand if you don't want to be obsessed with kilojoules, calories, fat grams or carbs. Even so, it is helpful information when you are first changing your diet, or investigating new foods. Becoming aware of the kilojoule content of the foods you eat will help you to make informed choices about your diet. It gives you a fresh perspective, and makes you realise that smaller portions, avoiding high-kilojoule beverages that don't fill you up, and keeping track of your fat and alcohol intake is important. Controlling your kilojoule intake puts you in the best position to burn off the excess kilojoules already stored on your body as fat.

Day 12 – Move more

Start off slowly, so you don't become an exercise dropout

It's very common for people to start a new exercise program like a bull at a gate, only to give up a few weeks later.

High expectations and slow results are not a good mix. This drop-off in enthusiasm often results in a lot of unused gym memberships and exercise machines becoming dust collectors.

Living it

Don't go too hard, too early. Start exercising at a level where you feel comfortable. Train at a low intensity for 2–4 weeks so your muscles and ligaments can adjust to your new and increased level of activity. If your exercise is more intense than walking, make sure you include one or two rest days each week to help your body to recover, and keep your mind fresh. Listen to your body, and if you start to feel tired or lacking in motivation, take a day off. Don't just give up.

Day 13 tip – Motivation and mindset

Use short-term goals, and plan a path to your long-term goal

Short-term goals are like stepping stones to help you reach your destination. These are the specific actions, steps, behaviours, skills and thinking processes you will need for your outcome to eventuate. You have much more control over the process than you do over the results. Some examples of short-term goals are:

- Plan your meals for the next 7 days

- Drink water before eating breakfast, lunch and dinner
- Have 3 alcohol-free nights each week
- Use your dumbbells twice each week
- Add interval training (see day 66) to your walks once a week
- Walk for 5 days this week.

Living it

Write down your long-term goal on a piece of paper, and plan out how you will achieve that goal in steps. Then transfer those steps and tasks into your diary. Writing down your goals is a valuable part of the goal-setting process. The visual reminder helps to focus your attention on the things that matter. When you consider that around 95% of dieters fail to lose weight and keep it off, and only 5% of the population writes down their goals, this simple step could make a world of difference.

Day 14 tip – Good food

Cut back your kilojoule intake gradually

When you cut back your kilojoule intake, one unfortunate side effect is that your metabolic rate will slow down. Your body realises that less fuel is coming in, so it makes a few adjustments to conserve kilojoules. This is sometimes referred to as survival mode, as your body uses its own defense mechanism against starvation. While you can't prevent this response you can actively minimise it, and keep your metabolism firing along. Try to reduce your kilojoule intake in small steps instead of making massive changes. Studies have shown that a dramatic cut in kilojoule intake can slow down the metabolism by as much as 45%, while a more gradual restriction can cut your metabolic rate as little as 10%.

Living it

A gradual reduction in kilojoules over time encourages the body to slowly use up fat stores. A dramatic reduction in kilojoules forces the body to break down some muscle protein to make up the deficit, and slows down your metabolism. Try to cut back a little bit more each week over 1 or 2 months. It's also important to point out that physical activity can also help to minimise the drop in your metabolic rate when you reduce your kilojoule intake.

Day 15 tip – Move more

Don't be discouraged by a little muscle soreness

Exercise can trigger a feeling of pain and stiffness in your muscles the day after your activity. Its scientific name is delayed onset muscle soreness (DOMS) because the pain usually appears 24–48 hours after the activity. It happens because physical activity causes microscopic ruptures in your muscles and surrounding tissues. It's nothing to worry about, but the muscles need a few days to repair, and the pain will gradually dissipate. It's most likely to occur:

- during the first 2–4 days of a new exercise program (especially resistance training)
- when you've had a break from training for more than 2 weeks
- when you add new movements, variations, duration, activities or intensity to your routine.

Living it

Expect a little soreness for your first 4–6 workouts if you are just starting out. It's normal, and part of the transformation from inactivity to activity. It's definitely not an excuse to give up. Studies on the best way of alleviating DOMS have shown stretching immediately after your activity and light massage to be most effective. If you are still experiencing muscle soreness from a previous workout but want to do something, it's best to keep your intensity light, or do warm-up and some stretching instead. If your muscle soreness persists after 3–5 days, and doesn't seem to be easing, or is in fact getting worse, you may have suffered an injury. Consider seeing your doctor, or a physiotherapist for diagnosis and treatment.

Day 16 tip – Motivation and mindset

Don't be disappointed if you gain a little weight when you start out

This might sound like bad news, but it's actually good news. When you begin to change your lifestyle it's normal to gain 1–2 kilos of muscle. You might even gain a fraction more if you are just starting to perform resistance training (weights) for the first time, or if you haven't done it for a while. Your inactive muscles don't know what's hit them, as they try to load up with water and extra glucose to prepare themselves for this new exercise routine. If you use the scales to measure your success, you might feel disheartened because there is no change in your weight when, in fact, you are going great. Gaining muscle doesn't make you bigger – just firmer and heavier. It means you are getting stronger and fitter, and that's certainly not something to feel bad about.

Living it

Don't be disappointed if the scales haven't budged that much in the first week or two. I know you want reassurance that these changes are worthwhile, so it's helpful to be aware of what to expect. Don't give up when you should actually be celebrating the positive steps you have taken towards better health and a better body shape. Use other measures to gauge your progress.

Day 17 tip – Good food

Understand that all kilojoules are not created equal

I have encouraged you to eat fewer kilojoules; but it's not just the number of kilojoules you eat, it's where they come from. There are four different ways you can consume kilojoules:

- **Fat** – which has 38 kilojoules per gram
- **Alcohol** – which has 29 kilojoules per gram
- **Carbohydrates** – which have 17 kilojoules per gram
- **Protein** – which has 17 kilojoules per gram

Living it

People don't eat kilojoules; they eat food. But it helps to know that fat is the most kilojoule dense food, containing more than double the energy content of carbohydrates and protein. Fat kilojoules also have the greatest capacity for storage because the body is very effective at converting dietary fat into body fat. In comparison, it's much harder for your body to convert excess protein and carbohydrate into body fat. Your body can't convert alcohol into fat, but it must be used for fuel first, making the kilojoules you consume with alcohol much more likely to be stored. So watch your alcohol intake, and focus on low-fat protein and quality carbohydrates that give you maximum fullness per kilojoule.

Day 18 tip – Move more

Make sure your exercise program is the right FITT

When you exercise to achieve weight and fat loss, it is important to follow a few basic guidelines. These guidelines vary depending on what you hope to achieve. For example, your exercise strategy to achieve fat loss will be different to the exercise factors you'll need to manipulate to increase aerobic fitness or muscle toning. To achieve results you'll need to juggle the four components of exercise that make the acronym FITT:

- **Frequency** – the amount of times you exercise in a week-long period
- **Intensity** – a measure of how hard you need to exercise to make sure that your exercise is effective; some measures include heart rate and breathing rate, and these may vary during an exercise session
- **Time** – the duration of your activity
- **Type** – the type of activity that is most likely to be beneficial.

Living it

The table below summarises the FITT principle for weight and fat loss.

Exercise factors	For weight and fat loss
Frequency	5–7 times per week
Intensity	Light to moderate, light huffing and puffing, 50–65% of maximum heart rate for beginners, 65–85% for the more advanced; also good to vary intensity with intervals
Time	30–60 minutes; this can also be accumulated over the day, especially for beginners
Type	Rhythmic, continuous movements that involve large muscle groups, like walking and jogging

Day 19 tip – Motivation and mindset
Use a tape measure, not the scales, to track your progress

I am not a big fan of focusing on weight loss. I like to help people lose weight, as long as that weight loss is through fat loss. It's body fat that's flabby and uncomfortable and unhealthy. A little extra weight, as long as it's through better hydration or increased muscle density, can actually help you lose body fat. In the first 4–12 weeks of commencing an exercise program, you'll experience the fastest and most dramatic improvements in muscle density. Your muscles don't get bigger, but they weigh more as they store more glucose (which is stored with water) to fuel your new activity. So use a tape measure to track your progress, especially when you start to exercise more often.

Living it

Use the table below to track your progress, and set a date to reassess your progress 3, 6 or 12 months later.

Measurement (centimetres)	Date _/_/_	Future date _/_/_
Waist at belly button		
Bottom at the widest point		
Upper right arm (mid point)		
Upper left arm (mid point)		
Right thigh (just below bottom)		
Left thigh (just below bottom)		
Right calf, widest point		
Left calf, widest point		

Day 20 tip – Good food

Don't count calories (or kilojoules), but be aware

Let's face it, counting kilojoules isn't anybody's idea of a good time. I don't expect anyone to count kilojoules, but it is important to cut back on them. So to cut back, it does help to be aware of what's high and what's not.

Living it

Get to know the rough kilojoule content of the foods you eat regularly. You don't have to calculate exactly how many you've eaten every day, but try to eat mostly foods with a lower kilojoule content. You can also use the kilojoule content on food labels to compare similar products, and choose the lower kilojoule variety. After a while you'll have a pretty good knowledge base of the better food choices, and you'll only have to check the kilojoule content on any new or unusual foods you try. Portion size is also important because if you eat too many low-kilojoule foods, you won't get results. Counting kilojoules for a few days is also something you might consider doing if you feel like you have been making all the right choices but aren't seeing any results. Ultimately, the more water you drink, and the more water-rich vegetables you eat, the less you will have to worry about counting kilojoules.

Day 21 tip – Move more

Don't change your diet without exercising

If you go on a diet, or cut back your kilojoule intake without being physically active, you actually make it harder for yourself to get results. Consider these facts:

- You will be less likely to burn off fat as a fuel source
- Your metabolic rate will slow down
- Your body will be more likely to store fat after the diet
- Any weight lost without exercise is virtually guaranteed to return within 12 months.

Combining regular exercise and healthy eating is the best way to burn dietary fat, and remove existing stores of body fat. This was shown in a recent 13-week study comparing two groups of cyclists. Both groups exercised twice a week, but one group cut out 800 kilojoules a day, while the second group kept their diet the same but burnt off 800 kilojoules with extra exercise. Both groups lost similar amounts of visceral (internal) fat, but the extra exercise group lost more subcutaneous fat. This type of fat is just beneath the skin, making your arms, legs and tummy look flabby. It appears that more weight can be lost by increasing your activity levels rather than by cutting kilojoules.

Living it

Exercise helps maintain muscle tissue. Food changes on their own are much less effective than combining healthy eating with regular exercise.

Day 22 tip – Motivation and mindset

The 3-week stocktake. Have you made any new habits yet?

Your are now into the third week of your personal *Lighten Up* program. How are you going? Have you adopted any new behaviours yet? Have you modified or cut out any habits that were holding you back from losing weight? Research has shown that if an action is repeated for a minimum of 21 days, it is more likely to become a permanent habit.

Living it

Why not identify one thing you could do every day for the next 21 days that will accelerate your results. I call this a 21-day challenge. Choose something that will have a big impact on your health and your weight, and stick to it for 21 days. It might be to cut out alcohol, eat less chocolate, plan your meals or exercise every day. Whatever you choose, plan for yourself a non-food related reward when you make the 21 days.

Day 23 tip – Good food

Calculate your daily fat needs, and keep to your fat budget

When you are trying to improve the way you eat, it's helpful to know just how much fat you should be having. Cutting back on fat will help to reduce your kilojoule intake; however, the amount of fat you need varies depending on your gender, your health goals and your activity levels. You don't have to count your fat grams permanently, but it does pay to be aware of how much fat is in the foods you eat regularly. The table below is a good guide to your daily fat requirements, which is like your personal 'fat budget' for weight loss.

Age and gender	Daily grams of fat	Daily kilojoules
Sedentary women and older adults	35	5500
Teenage girls, active women and sedentary men	45	7000
Teenage boys, active men and extremely active women	53	8000

Living it

The fat budget is ideal in that it gives you endless options, and does not restrict the total amount of food you eat. You can still fill up on healthy vegetables, wholegrain cereals, fruits, legumes and whole grains, and stay within your fat budget. It also helps you to balance how much fat you get from packaged foods, which is often listed as fat grams per serving on the nutrition information panel. Your personal fat budget can be increased or decreased by 5–10 grams depending on your frame size and how much fat you have to lose. Just try to make sure that the majority of fats you eat are healthy plant fats.

Day 24 tip – Move more

Set a benchmark, and test your cardiovascular fitness

To get anywhere, you need to know your starting place. When it comes to starting an exercise program for weight loss, that means giving yourself a basic fitness assessment. Yes, the focus of this book is fat loss, not fitness, but improved cardiovascular fitness will improve your ability to burn fat. This is not about proving you are unfit; it will help to you measure your progress and motivate you to improve.

Living it

One of the easiest tests you can do is a timed walk or run over a set distance. You can do this on a treadmill, or map out a set course using your car odometer. Aim for a distance of 3–5 kilometres depending on your weight and level of fitness. The main thing is that this distance or course needs to be repeated in the future. Once you've completed the test, cool down, and then write down your results below. I'm not going to give you a score or ranking because the only person you are competing against is yourself. We will re-test you again later to evaluate your improvement.

Warning – Unless you are already in pretty good condition, don't push yourself to get a really good time. If you feel any chest pain or discomfort, stop the test immediately. Just work at a comfortable pace, and work within your limits.

Date	
Course distance/description	
Time to completion	
Heart rate 60 seconds after completion (optional)	

Day 25 tip – Motivation and mindset

Check to see if excess body fat is affecting your health

How's your waist management? What was your waist circumference from day 19. If your waist measurement is too large, your current level of body fat is placing your health at risk. Excess fat stored around your stomach can point towards heart disease, and has been closely linked with breast cancer and insulin resistance in women and colon cancer and diabetes in men. Abdominal fat can also be a major cause of snoring and high blood pressure. Measure your waist around the navel and use the table below to assess your level of health risk.

Health risk	Low	Medium	High
Women's waist	less than 80cm	80–90cm	91cm or more
Men's waist	less than 90cm	90–100cm	101cm or more

A measurement of more than 90cm in men and 80cm in women doubles your chances of having one or more of the risk factors for heart disease. A waist circumference of more than 101cm in men and 91cm in women indicates you are overweight and should reduce body fat before health problems occur. Fortunately, abdominal fat stores respond best to lifestyle changes.

Living it

Waist measurement is a good way to check if you really need to do something about your current level of body fat. It can be motivating to have a target, especially one that's more relevant and accurate than total body weight.

Day 26 tip – Good food

Know which fat is which

All fats are not created equal. While all types are high in kilojoules and should be eaten in moderation for weight loss, some types are better for your health than others. The three main types of dietary fat found in foods are saturated, polyunsaturated and mono-unsaturated. Mono-unsaturated fats provide the best protection against heart disease. Saturated fat is considered the dietary bad guy because of its negative effect on your blood cholesterol levels. Polyunsaturated fats tend to have a neutral effect on your cholesterol, except for foods containing processed polyunsaturated fats called trans fats. Trans fats are just as harmful to your health as saturated fats and are common in margarine and fast foods.

Living it

Try to get most of your fat intake from mono-unsaturated fats and unprocessed polyunsaturated fats. Minimise your intake of saturated fats, and processed polyunsaturated fats (trans fats).

Mono-unsaturated	Polyunsaturated	Saturated
Olive oil, peanuts, peanut oil, canola oil, avocado, oily fish (salmon, tuna), macadamia oil, lean meats	Safflower, sunflower, corn, sesame, soybean and grape seed oils, margarine, fish, shellfish, sunflower and pumpkin seeds, walnuts, brazil nuts, pine nuts	Butter, cheese, beef and chicken fat, palm oil, cakes, vegetable shortening, pastries, coconut cream, chocolate, hydrogenated vegetable oil, carob, copha

Day 27 tip – Move more

Do more incidental movement

Can you believe that lots of little bits of movement throughout the day can burn kilojoules and actually help you lose weight? While it's not as effective as structured exercise, any extra activity helps; and it doesn't have to be vigorous. Random acts of movement are a good way to counteract deskwork, inactive leisure time, and labour-saving technology that has dramatically reduced the amount of kilojoules we use every day.

Living it

Look for ways to incorporate more movement into your lifestyle, and not for ways to avoid it. Any extra movement is an opportunity to burn extra kilojoules, which can also help to make your planned exercise more effective.

- When you can, walk instead of using your car.
- Use the stairs instead of lifts or escalators.
- Get off public transport before your stop and walk the rest of the way.
- Park your car some distance from your destination and walk.
- Walk to the next office rather than emailing a co-worker.
- Go for a short walk during your lunch break.

Day 28 tip – Motivation and mindset

Identify the barriers to your success

Why can't you lose weight? What is holding you back from getting results? Here are some of the more common limiting factors or underlying barriers to weight and fat loss:

- drinking too much alcohol, or other empty kilojoules
- eating too much takeaway food
- eating large portion sizes, especially at night
- excessive TV viewing
- lack of exercise and physical activity
- overeating due to stress or emotional issues
- eating too many processed carbohydrates.

Living it

As long as these barriers remain unidentified they will continue to stop you from getting results. Think about your lifestyle and your diet. Honestly evaluate yourself. Ask yourself what's working and what's not. Do you have problem areas that are holding you back? Ask a close friend to tell you honestly what they think is holding you back. What three changes could you make that would make the biggest difference to your health and wellness? Think about your answers and you'll discover what limiting factors are stopping you from losing weight. Hopefully, it will then become clear what you need to change.

Day 29 tip – Good food

To cut back on fat, find out where it comes from

Cutting down on fat is one of the most effective ways to reduce your kilojoule intake and accelerate weight loss. Dietary fat usually comes from three main sources:

Where fat comes from	Examples	Comments
Fats occurring naturally in foods	meats, nuts, butter, cheese, whole milk, yoghurt, avocado	Trim visible fats from meats, choose low-fat dairy products
Fats you add during cooking	butter, cooking oils, eggs, salad dressings, cream	Cut back, or substitute healthier ingredients
Fats manufactured with foods	cakes, biscuits, snack foods, pastry, chocolate	Cat back as much as you can, look for low-fat alternatives

Living it

Have a look at the table above and see where you can make changes to reduce your fat intake. Although it will help to cut back on all fats, try to minimise your intake of the manufactured fats, which tend to be the worst choice for your heart, and your waist. When you do eat fat, eat fats that are the least processed, especially the plant fats found in nuts, seeds, avocado and olive oil.

Day 30 tip – Move more

Don't be embarrassed to exercise

Do you hate the thought of exercising in public? Embarrassment is recognised as one of the main reasons people avoid physical activity. It can stem from a fear of looking silly, or negative experiences from the past that foster a negative attitude towards exercise. Some of this fear of embarrassment is associated with gyms, where people feel uncomfortable in that environment or intimidated by being around people who are in good shape. Other reasons may be that people feel too old or unskilled to operate equipment, lack co-ordination or worry they won't be able to keep up in classes. Some even fear they'll destroy the equipment. This becomes a vicious cycle, where the people who need to exercise more are the ones most likely to feel uncomfortable doing it. But you don't have to join a gym or play sports to be active. However, you will have to be active if you are serious about losing body fat.

Living it

It's important to feel relaxed and comfortable when you exercise. If you feel embarrassed exercising in public, look at ways you can exercise at home. Get some exercise equipment or an instructional video, or even try walking at night (wearing brightly coloured clothing). As your fitness improves and you lose weight, your confidence will grow and any embarrassment will be less of an issue.

Day 31 tip – Motivation and mindset

Have a plan to overcome the barriers that are holding you back

The barriers that stop people from losing weight are often learned and habitual. Being able to see these barriers is an important step in addressing them. When you have a better understanding of the habits and attitudes that are holding you back, you'll be in the best position make a plan to do something about them.

Living it

Whatever your barriers are, here are some problem-solving strategies to address, replace or remove them.

- **Anticipate** – Think about the situations or surroundings where your barriers arise. What can you do to prevent them from occurring? For example, if you drink too much socially, you can offer to drive.

- **Break it down into smaller chunks** – Some barriers are simply too big to break down all at once, like emotional eating. Start to manage the pieces bit by bit and it becomes more achievable. For example, start by looking at how to deal with stress in other ways, and once you make some progress, look at limiting the junk foods you have around the house.

- **Turn it to your advantage** – A little creativity can turn your barriers into supporters. For example, if you watch too much TV, use your time constructively and buy a treadmill so you can work out at the same time.

- **Give yourself time** – These barriers may have been with you for a while, like eating large portions at night. Try to whittle down your portion size gradually instead of making drastic changes you can't stick to.

Day 32 tip – Good food

Be patient with your taste buds. Train them well

When you first cut back on sugar, salt or fat, your taste buds may not appreciate it. They expect the flavours and textures of foods they come in contact with most often. But your taste buds renew themselves every few weeks. Think of someone you know who has cut sugar out of their tea. It's generally tough for a few weeks, but then it gets easier, and after a while they can enjoy tea without sugar. They might even be able to tell if sugar was on the spoon used to stir their tea. The same applies to cutting back on fat, such as switching from full-cream milk to skim milk, or using less butter on your toast.

Living it

Give yourself a month for your taste buds to adjust to a different way of eating. You may even need a little longer if you are over 70 years of age when the taste buds are less sensitive. Stay patient, use herbs and spices to add flavour without fat, and train your taste buds to enjoy healthier eating.

Day 33 tip – Move more

If you walk for weight loss, follow these five steps

If you had to pick one activity that is best for weight loss, and suits the majority of people, walking is a clear stand out. It's an easy, accessible and enjoyable way to lose weight, get fit, reduce stress and boost your energy levels. It can be done almost anywhere, anytime, by anyone, and best of all – it's free. But walking is actually a very easy, efficient activity for your body, and doesn't burn a lot of kilojoules, especially if you just cruise along. Studies have shown that up to 94% of walkers don't walk frequently enough or fast enough to gain real health benefits.

Living it

Following are 5 key strategies that can help you make walking a more effective, fat-burning exercise.

- **Walk fast** – Speed matters. People who maintain a faster pace while walking will burn more kilojoules and get better results. Try to swing your arms, and walk as if you're 5 minutes late.

- **Walk long** – When you are just starting out, any walking is ideal. But after a month or two, longer walks will bring you better results. Aim for around 3–4 hours of walking every 7 days. See day 36 for more details.

- **Walk often** – Aim for 4–7 days a week, depending on how fast and for how long you walk. Try not to miss 2 days in a row of cardiovascular exercise.

- **Step it up as you get fitter** – The more you walk, the more efficient your body gets at moving you around. To keep burning more and more kilojoules, up the duration, intensity or frequency of your walks as your fitness improves. You will learn more about this later.

- **Mix it up** – Add variety to your routine by walking on different surfaces (grass, sand, hills), at different times of the day, for different durations, at different intensities (interval training is a must) or intersperse some body weight exercises (push-ups, lunges) along the way.

Day 34 tip – Motivation and mindset

Know why you want to lose weight

It might seem obvious, but it really helps to have a clear understanding of the reasons why you want to shed body fat. You will have a better chance of achieving your goals if you are truly convinced of the benefits that your new behaviours will bring. This can help to inspire you and keep you on track during times of doubt. Some of the more common positive reasons people want to lose weight include to improve your health, buy new clothes, or fit back into old clothes, improve your appearance, feel more confident at a special event, improve your fitness level, have more energy, or to sleep better.

Living it

It's important to know what you want out of a healthy lifestyle and focus on how the changes you make will improve your quality of life. Write down, or at the very least identify in your mind, two positive things you want from reducing your level of stored body fat. You can write these two points on the lines below, and remind yourself of them when you are struggling for motivation. You could call these your change motivators.

1. ....

2. ....

Day 35 tip – Good food

Forget about low fat on its own. It simply won't work

You won't lose a lot of weight eating low-fat biscuits or ice-cream. Low fat is so nineties, so make sure you're not living in the past. What happened was that people ate low-fat foods like bread, pasta and rice without guilt or moderation in the belief that anything without fat was open slather. And people didn't get great results. In fact, some just got fatter. Unfortunately, the accompanying message to eat high fibre or exercise more never seemed to generate the same attention or hysteria. Nutritional research and exercise science has also come a long way since then and we now know the importance of the glycogenic index, energy density, reducing sugar, portion size, healthy fats and interval training.

Living it

Of course, eating less fat is a useful strategy for weight and fat loss because high-fat foods are high-kilojoule foods. But unless you combine a low-fat diet with other strategies like portion control, a high fibre intake, regular exercise, moderating your alcohol intake and including some healthy fats, you will struggle to get results.

Day 36 tip – Move more

Walk more than 15 minutes a day

Walking is a great exercise for fat loss, but it is an easy activity that doesn't burn a lot of kilojoules, so you need to do plenty of it to get results. For example, one study showed that walking briskly for 15 minutes each day is not enough to burn off the extra kilojoules in most people's diet. It was recommended that people walk briskly for an average of 30 minutes each day, or 60 minutes if they prefer a slower pace.

Living it

While any exercise is better than none when you are first starting out, you will need to walk briskly for more than 15 minutes a day if you want life changing, body shape changing results. The chart below helps you look at things from a 7-day perspective, where you can vary your duration based on your frequency. You can also reduce your total duration by doing more kilojoule intensive exercise like jogging.

Frequency	Slow walking	Brisk walking	Jogging
4 days a week	120 minutes	60 minutes	30 minutes
5 days a week	100 minutes	50 minutes	25 minutes
6 days a week	80 minutes	40 minutes	20 minutes
7 days a week	60 minutes	30 minutes	15 minutes

Day 37 tip – Motivation and mindset

Check on your attitude towards change

There are some challenges that everyone must face when making changes, and choosing to get lean and healthy. That's why it's so important to be aware of your attitude and level of commitment before you start.

Living it

Put your attitude to the test, and answer these questions to find out if you are in the right frame of mind to succeed at long-term weight and fat loss.

1. Do you believe that health and body fat reduction is a major priority in your life at the moment?

2. Do you have confidence in your ability to make lifestyle changes at this point in your life?

3. Can you accept the idea that permanent, not temporary changes to

your eating habits and activity levels are needed for you to be successful?

4. Can you accept the idea that it is best to lose body fat gradually and focus on the long-term?

5. Do you have a positive attitude about being more active and a willingness to include more movement in your life?

6. Do you have a positive attitude about eating more healthily and a willingness to commit more time towards planning for and preparing healthier foods?

I hope you had mostly yes answers to the questions above. The more 'no' answers you had, the harder it is going to be for you to stick with your lifestyle changes. You may not be ready to make changes, or you might need to learn more about some of those factors before commencing. You would be better off dealing with some emotional issues first, or seeking the help of a personal trainer or dietician to help kick-start the process.

Day 38 tip – Good food

Drink lots of water (and don't ignore this tip)

Do you drink 6–8 glasses of water every day? A lot of people know they should, but don't. It's a well-known weight-loss tip and here's why.

- **It reduces your kilojoule intake** – Drinking water instead of soft drinks, fruit juice, cordial, sports drinks and alcohol can help to significantly reduce your kilojoule intake.

- **It prevents hunger** – Water is a natural appetite suppressant; however, thirst is not a reliable guide to your body's fluid needs. A lack of water can actually make you hungry. By drinking enough water, you can help to prevent hunger.

- **It helps your metabolism** – Water is needed to metabolise or break down stored fats. It is also needed for other metabolic functions like digestion, food absorption and regulation of body temperature.

- **It prevents food cravings** – Drinking water regularly helps to cleanse your taste buds of flavours that might otherwise trigger a food craving.

Living it

Try to drink a few glasses of chilled water before breakfast, lunch and dinner. The extra fullness will help to reduce your kilojoule intake, and boost your metabolic rate. Have a little extra if it's hot, if it's humid, if you participate in strenuous exercise, when you drink lots of caffeine or alcohol, or if you work in an air-conditioned office.

Day 39 tip – Move more

Try shorter, more frequent exercise sessions

Is it difficult for you to find the time to exercise? One solution is to accumulate your exercise over the course of the day. Research suggests that breaking exercise sessions into smaller segments can still have significant benefits. A study compared two groups; one who did 40 minutes of exercise in one hit, another who accumulated their 40 minutes in four, 10-minute sessions throughout the day. The women who exercised for shorter periods were more likely to stick with their exercise program. They often exercised for more than the prescribed 5 days per week and accumulated more than 40 minutes. A similar study showed that a short bout group lost 40% more weight, although this is more likely to be a result of their extra exercise and not because the short bouts are more effective at burning fat.

Living it

If you are very busy, are looking after small children or feel like trying something new, why not accumulate your exercise over the day. If you are just beginning an exercise program, short bouts are just as effective for weight loss. However, as your fitness improves, perform your exercise continuously for increased fat burning.

Day 40 tip – Motivation and mindset

Embrace the changes you need to make

The reality about losing body fat is that you must step out of your comfort zone and make changes to your current eating and activity habits if you want to succeed. For some people, change itself is harder to deal with than being fat, and they will stay fat. But change is your ticket to better quality and quantity of life, so why not focus on what it can do for you, instead of worrying about how hard it is.

Living it

Making real changes is what will bring you real results, so embrace the changes you make. A positive attitude can make all the difference. Until you adopt a different approach, you won't break the cycle. You won't get results until you think, move and eat differently.

Day 41 tip – Good food

Develop a good understanding of the glycemic index

Don't let the technical name turn you off. The glycemic Index, or GI, is a great weight-loss tool because it ranks carbohydrate foods based on how fast they raise your blood glucose levels. The GI is much more accurate than calling carbohydrates simple or complex. For example, white rice (thought of as a complex carbohydrate) is absorbed faster than honey (known as a simple carbohydrate). Foods that release glucose slowly (low GI foods) are much more likely to fill you up, while foods that release glucose quickly (high GI foods) give you a sudden burst of energy but can leave you tired and hungry soon after. Low GI foods also reduce the need for insulin.

Living it

Low GI diets help with weight loss because they make you feel full with less kilojoules. Try to include more low GI food in your diet.

Low GI foods	Medium GI foods	High GI foods
Rice bran, yoghurt, skim milk, grain and rye bread, barley, wholegrain pasta, chickpeas, oranges, soy-beans, lentils, tomatoes, porridge, All-Bran and cherries	Sustain, Basmati rice, white bread, wholemeal bread, banana, soft drinks, cordial, orange juice, popcorn, muesli bars, pasta, baked beans	Puffed wheat, Rice Bub-bles, cornflakes, Calrose rice, bagel, pumpkin, jelly beans, watermelon, car-rots, potatoes, corn chips, croissants, ice-cream

Day 42 tip – Move more

Try not to miss 2 days in a row of exercise

How much exercise is enough? Until recently, it was thought that 20 minutes of physical exercise three times a week was all that was needed for good health and weight control. While anything is better than nothing, we now know that this is not enough to derive health benefits let alone significant weight loss. To lose weight you need to send a consistent message to your fat cells that they are not needed. If you can exercise at least 4 days a week, that means you are active more than 50% of the time. If you can exercise more, that will send an even stronger message that your body can adapt to. By exercising every day, or at least every second day, you will increase your chances of getting results.

Living it

Do your best to exercise 4–7 days each week to maximise your chances of getting results. Avoid missing 2 days in a row of exercise.

Day 43 tip – Motivation and mindset

Find your own light bulb moment

The information on motivation and mindset throughout *Lighten Up* is designed to address the most underestimated issue in changing your lifestyle and losing weight – your thoughts and attitude. They way you think about and approach weight loss will make a big difference to your results. A lot of people have the knowledge but don't act on it. A lot of people want to lose weight but don't do anything about it. A lot of people read a lot of diet books but haven't lost weight or kept it off. So how is this book different?

Living it

This book is different because of you – the reader. Somewhere in these pages you'll find a few short words, a sentence, a thought or a new way of looking at things that helps you see everything from a new perspective. It might be the culmination of several tips that allows you to make changes and succeed at prioritising your health. You could call it a light bulb moment, where things suddenly become clear about why you have to make changes and why you can make it work this time. If you look hard enough, you'll find it. I hope you do.

Day 44 tip – Good food

Enjoy alcohol in moderation, and have MAD days

If you enjoy a drink, I've got mixed news. The good news is that you don't need to eliminate alcohol to lose weight. If it's something you enjoy then you can continue to have alcohol in moderation. In fact, I encourage it. There's no point depriving yourself, as it only makes you want it more. Just try to limit yourself to 1–2 small drinks on the days you do indulge. But the reality you must face is that if you drink a little every day, or if you binge drink, you will find it very difficult, if not impossible, to lose body fat. If you are serious about losing weight and fat, you should aim for 3–5 alcohol-free days each week. These are called MAD days, which stands for 'Miss A Day'. If the thought of a MAD day seems … well, madness to you, try to balance out your alcohol intake with other strategies. Consider the following:

- drinking less than you are now
- spacing out your drinks with a glass of water

- drinking low alcohol or reduced alcohol drinks
- using low-kilojoule mixers
- doing extra exercise
- eating very well on the days that you drink.

Living it

If you drink alcohol, try to have less than you currently do to help cut down your kilojoule intake, or look for other ways to compensate. Try to have at least three alcohol-free (MAD) days each week.

Day 45 tip – Move more

Don't be discouraged by statements like 'no pain, no gain'

Are you discouraged by the fact that exercise is meant to hurt to be beneficial? Don't worry. 'No pain no gain' does not apply when you start exercising to burn fat. If you are a beginner, or feel like you are unfit, focus on rhythmic, continuous movement like walking to burn fat. Intense exercise such as interval training does have its benefits, but that's something you can build up to. As your fitness improves, and your tolerance for exercise increases, you can up the intensity without too much discomfort. It's important to point out that the exercise intensity required to burn fat is different to what's required to get super fit or add muscle bulk through heavy weight training. These different goals require you to push your body to its limits to get results, and experience what most people would perceive as pain.

Living it

Begin gradually, and let your body adapt to exercise over a month or two. Then begin to up the ante by going a little faster, training longer or getting active a little more often. If your progress is steady and gradual, you can get great results without pain. As your fitness improves you'll need to exert yourself to a point of mild discomfort to continue to improve. But your body will be prepared, and you may even enjoy the feeling.

Day 46 tip – Motivation and mindset

Reward yourself for adopting new lifestyle habits

Do you have an incentive or way to reward yourself for any new lifestyle changes you have adopted? When you've reached a goal, whether small or large, give yourself a treat. Knowing there is a reward to be gained reinforces your healthy behaviour and helps to drive you towards taking action. It can be especially helpful for those times when you really don't feel like it and just want to revert back to your old ways. Make sure your goals are challenging yet do-able, and that the rewards match the task. You can choose to reward yourself weekly, fortnightly or monthly – whatever makes you feel good. Use little rewards for your smaller goals, and larger rewards when you achieve your long-term goals. Make sure you also include rewards that focus on the process, not just the results, such as walking 6 days each week or keeping your portions small at night. Finally, choose non-food related rewards that won't blow all your good work, such as getting a massage or buying a new book or CD.

Living it

Find a unique reward system that motivates you, especially when you are starting out. As your new lifestyle changes become habits, you can make your rewards more distant and harder to achieve, as your new level of health and wellness becomes a reward in itself.

Day 47 tip – Good food

Keep your portion size under control

Do you eat pretty well but struggle to lose weight? It's possible you are eating too much. Portion size is vital for weight control because the bigger your serving, the bigger your kilojoule intake. Studies show that most people eat more than the recommended serving sizes for many foods, with an estimated 600 additional kilojoules consumed today beyond the average from just 20 years ago. People also tend to eat what's put in front of them. One study showed that when two groups had access to unlimited lasagna, the group who first received a large portion ate more than the group who were first given a small portion, even though both groups were allowed to get up for more.

Living it

Following are some strategies to help reduce your portion sizes and get the maximum fullness from your foods with the least amount of kilojoules.

- **Slow down** – People who eat slower tend to eat less.
- **Eat well** – Unprocessed foods are absorbed slowly, making you feel fuller for longer.
- **Drink water** – Water can fill your stomach and take the edge off hunger.
- **Eat less, more often** – Spread your kilojoule intake over the day.

- **Use the 10-minute rule** – Wait 10 minutes if you ever want seconds; the craving may pass.

Day 48 tip – Move more

If you are trying to convince yourself that you don't need to exercise today, remember this

There will always be days when you don't feel like training, but remember that exercise can do a lot more than help you to lose weight. The benefits include a stronger heart and lungs, increased bone density, reduced risk of heart disease and cancer, and increased longevity. That's all well and good, but it's hard to get motivated by things that take time to materialise. This is why it helps to focus on what exercise can do for you today. Even just 10 minutes can offer benefits, and once you actually start, you might even feel like doing a little more. That's why they say that the hardest part is just putting on your exercise gear. Once you are actually out there moving, you can almost guarantee you'll feel better for it or feel glad that you did it when you've finished.

Living it

If you ever experience days that you don't feel like exercising, bookmark this page and check out what exercise can do for you today:

- Makes you feel more energetic and revitalised
- Lowers mental and muscular tension
- Helps you feel good about yourself, knowing you have done something today to achieve your health and fat loss goals
- Shows your new level of resolve, that this time you will get the results you seek
- Improves your ability to fall asleep and sleep well
- Increases your ability to concentrate and think faster.

Day 49 tip – Motivation and mindset

Solve your own weight-loss puzzle

One of the best ways to describe weight loss and emphasise how it's different for every person, is to compare it to a jigsaw puzzle. There are 30 to 40 pieces that all need to work together to make everything fall into place. There is no single cure. Some people may have their food all sorted out but struggle to get their exercise together. Others are okay with exercise but drink too much alcohol. Every person is different and may need to focus on different aspects of their weight-loss puzzle to get the picture right.

Food-related parts of the puzzle	Activity-related parts of the puzzle	Other parts to the puzzle
Fat intake	Activity in the workplace	Genetics and biology
Fat type	Transport to/from work	Stress
Portion size	Planned activity	Medication
Protein quality	Incidental activity	Disease and illness (thyroid)
Energy density	Type of activity	Age
Glycemic index (carb quality)	Intensity of activity	History of crash dieting
Food variety	Duration of activity	Gender
Levels of hunger	Frequency of activity	Fear of failure
Night eating	Fatigue or laziness	Pregnancy/menopause
Binge eating	Injury/incapacity	Smoking cessation
Social/holiday eating	Childhood experiences	Environment
No hunger eating	Metabolism	Motivation and willpower
Comfort eating	Post-exercise exhaustion/ soreness	Fear of crime
Alcohol	Self-consciousness during exercise	Weather
Food intake with alcohol	Muscle mass/strength	Family commitments

Living it

As you work through *Lighten Up*, and we address these issues over time, try to develop an awareness of the pieces of the puzzle you need to work on. You'll then be in the best position to do something about it.

Day 50 tip – Good food

Fill up on fibre

Dietary fibre is vital for health and weight control, yet most Australians only consume around half their daily fibre needs. Research has shown that increasing your fibre intake can reduce the absorption of fat from other foods. Volunteers doubled their daily fibre intake to 36 grams, reducing the absorption of fat in their diet by up to 131 calories (550 kilojoules). Fibre can also help you lose weight because it fills you up, it's low in kilojoules, it decreases the room for fatty foods and it improves control of your blood sugar levels (requiring less insulin).

Living it

Fibre can only be found in plant foods; it's recommended that adults consume 30 grams a day. Here are some ways you can increase your fibre intake:

- Have a bran-based, high fibre breakfast cereal
- Sprinkle wheatgerm, wheat bran, oat bran, barely bran or rice bran on your breakfast cereal
- Substitute some of the meat in meals with extra vegetables and/or some of the large varieties of legumes
- Choose wholegrain or wholemeal options for bread, flour, rice and pasta
- Try to snack on high fibre foods like baked beans, fruit and breakfast cereals
- Eat the skins of fruit and vegetables like carrots, potatoes, apples and pears.

Day 51 tip – Move more

Maximise you metabolic rate

Metabolism is a collective term for all the functions going on in your body that you don't even think about, like your digestion, breathing, circulation and tissue repair. Organs such as your stomach, lungs, heart and brain all use kilojoules to keep you alive, even when you sleep. Metabolic rate is the variable speed at which your body uses kilojoules for your metabolism, and this is why some people use more kilojoules for their metabolism than others. It's like the engine in a car: if you rev it up it uses more fuel, but if you let it idle on low it uses less fuel. A faster, revved up metabolic rate is vital for weight control, helping you burning more kilojoules, not just while you're active but also while you're resting.

Living it

There are some key strategies you can use to rev up your engine and get your metabolism firing.

- **Exercise** – Exercise is like pressing the accelerator in your car, making your engine function quicker and burn more fuel. Extra energy is used both during and after exercise.
- **Get strong** – Muscles demand lots of kilojoules. Resistance training protects and even increases the density of muscle (not necessarily the size), helping to boost your metabolic rate.
- **Don't starve** – If your kilojoule intake is too low, your metabolic rate

will slow down as a survival mechanism and conserve stored body fat. A little hunger is okay, but don't starve.

- **Eat breakfast** – First thing in the morning your body hasn't had any fuel for 8–12 hours. Breakfast is vital to kick-start your metabolic rate for the day.
- **Others** – Spicy foods, smaller but more frequent eating, cold temperatures, raw foods, caffeine and eating a wide variety of nutritious foods all have a metabolism boosting effect.

Day 52 tip – Motivation and mindset

Identify the consequences of inaction (if you don't lose weight)

While some people will be motivated enough to seek out the positive benefits that come from making lifestyle changes, others need a little bit more of a push. Some people need a bit of a scare, some straight talk from their doctor or the illness of a friend to shock them into action. Thinking about what will happen to you if you don't lose weight may be enough to motivate you.

Living it

Just as it is a choice to take action and make changes, it is also a choice to wait till a later time. Thinking about the consequences of your inaction may be enough to help spark a fire that gets you started. What do you fear most if you don't change your lifestyle? How is excess body fat holding you back? What are the things you miss out on, what are you not achieving, what activities do you avoid? How will you look and feel in 1, 2 or 5 years' time if you don't change your lifestyle? How will you feel in 12 months' time looking back at this moment, knowing you had an opportunity to do something and did nothing? Maybe you are on the edge of developing diabetes or heart disease, or feel worried that you won't be able to keep up with your kids. Write down at least two things that worry you, or that may happen to you if you don't lose weight. Then keep your answers to these questions close by for those times when you might need a quick reality check on why you are making changes.

1. ....

2. ....

Day 53 tip – Good food

Make your vegetables water rich and less starchy

We all know that vegetables are healthy, but did you know there are some types that are nearly 10 times more likely to help you get results. Fibrous, or water-rich vegetables have a low kilojoule content because they have a high percentage of water and fibre per gram. They can still fill you up, but have around 10 times less kilojoules per serving than starchy vegetables. For a complete list of the different types of vegetables, see the table below.

Water-rich vegetables	Starchy vegetables
Asparagus, broccoli, cabbage, cauliflower, zucchini, capsicum, mushrooms, onions, tomatoes, green beans, alfalfa, bamboo shoots, spinach, leeks, chili, squash, celery, eggplant, brussels sprouts, bok choy, snow peas, spring onions, artichokes, fennel, lettuce, carrots, baby corn, cucumber **Aim for 4–5* servings per day**	Potato, corn, pumpkin, peas and sweet potato **Aim for 1* serving per day**
Eg celery (100 grams) = 50kJ	Eg potato (100g) = 400kJ

* 1 serving is enough to fill half a cup

Living it

Make water-rich vegetables the foundation of your evening meal. Try different types of vegetables regularly, or vary your cooking methods, such as steamed, sautéed, baked, stir-fried or grilled. Have them as main course, as a snack or in a soup or side dish.

Day 54 tip – Move more

Generate momentum for your exercise program

How consistent are you with your exercise? Getting on a roll can help you get results and be motivating. The principle of momentum implies that while it may take a lot of effort to get started, it then takes far less effort to keep going. For example, when you start to exercise, you'll feel better about yourself, which makes you want to eat a little better; and when you lose a little fat, you'll find exercise a little easier, which motivates you a little more. The further you go, the more experience you get and the more you learn. You also become more confident, and your self-belief and self-esteem grows.

Living it

Identify a few small changes you could make (like walking every day for a week) and try to start a small roll, even if it's for a short time. This will breed confidence and put you back on track, helping to build momentum.

Day 55 tip – Motivation and mindset

Be accountable to someone

Having someone who is checking on your progress can really make a difference to your motivation. To get a little outside support, you might need to go public and make your weight-loss attempt well known. Even better, find someone who is also making lifestyle changes and you can keep track of each other.

Living it

Who are you accountable to? You can be accountable to yourself, although being accountable to others is usually a stronger source of motivation. Being accountable is a vital component of weight loss, and you will find more information on all the following strategies throughout *Lighten Up*.

- **You** – Use a food diary, exercise journal, commitment contract or quarterly monthly measurements to be accountable to yourself.

- **Others** – Report to a partner, friend, training buddy, work colleague, personal trainer, online weight-loss coach, weight-loss support group, exercise group or web blog.

Day 56 tip – Good food

Always eat breakfast

Do you eat breakfast every day? A good breakfast has long been recommended for weight and fat loss, yet research shows it is the meal most people skip. Breakfast is associated with:

- improved energy, strength and endurance
- prevention of hunger and mid-morning food cravings
- elevation of your metabolic rate
- mental alertness and a positive attitude towards the day.

Studies have also shown that a high fibre breakfast helps to reduce the total amount of kilojoules you eat for the rest of the day. If you don't feel like breakfast, it's possible the portion size of your evening meal is too large.

Living it

If you are determined to reduce body fat, you should try to eat breakfast every day. Cut back on your portion size at night and you will feel hungry in the morning.

Day 57 tip – Move more

Eat less on inactive days, and don't eat more on active days

One of the keys to losing weight is to adjust your kilojoule intake to match your activity levels. You could call this the 'adjust as you go' strategy. It's also important to listen to your body, and try to become more aware of how physical activity, or the lack of it, affects your hunger levels.

Living it

There are two key strategies that help you 'adjust as you go'.

- **Eat less when you're inactive** – You probably won't be able to exercise every day of the week. That's fine, but you won't be burning off as many kilojoules on the days you don't exercise, so try not to eat as many. You can drop off a snack, reduce your portion size, eliminate alcohol, and drink more water to maximise fullness.

- **Don't eat more on the days you do exercise** – Following exercise you'll probably have low blood sugar levels (especially if you exercise when you're hungry). While this will help you to burn more fat, be aware that low blood sugar levels can trigger a sensation of hunger that is greater than your actual kilojoule needs. Drink plenty of water afterwards, delay your eating as long as possible, and eat slowly when you do eat.

Day 58 tip – Motivation and mindset

Commit yourself to a better body (contractually)

Even with all the knowledge in the world, it's ultimately your motivation and level of commitment that will determine your success. One way of keeping yourself accountable is to write a commitment contract to yourself. You then have a written record of exactly what you want, why you want it, and what you'll miss out on if you don't get it.

Living it

Make a commitment to your new, healthier lifestyle by putting it in writing. Take a blank piece of paper and write out the following:

- Your long-term goal (see day 10 for ideas)
- Two reasons why you'd like to achieve your goal (add what you wrote down on day 34)
- Two things you fear about not achieving your goal (add what you wrote down on day 52)
- I hereby commit to (write down at least two of the following, or add your own):
  - Making health and fitness a priority in my life
  - Not letting slip ups defeat me
  - Looking for solutions to becoming healthier; not making excuses
  - Call on others to support me while I try to achieve my goals
  - Not letting outside influences interfere with my determination to achieve my goals
  - Not using food to help deal with any problems or stress
- Sign and date it.

Once it's signed, stick it on your fridge to as a daily reminder. If not, at least read through and think about the level of commitment you are prepared to make towards a healthier life.

Day 59 tip – Good food

Five simple breakfast swaps to make those kilos drop

A few small dietary changes can make a big difference over time. Eating an extra 200 kilojoules takes around 10 minutes of moderate walking to burn off, so every little bit counts.

Living it

Here are five small things you can do at breakfast to reduce your fat and kilojoule intake and accelerate your weight loss.

Instead of...	Go for...	Save...	Comments
Fruit juice (250ml) = 440 kilojoules	Tomato juice (250ml) = 200 kilojoules	240 kilojoules	While water is best, tomato juice has less than half the kilojoules of fruit juice, and a lower GI
1 croissant and butter = 1125 kilojoules	English muffin with jam = 700 kilojoules	425 kilojoules	The muffin has more fibre, and will be far more filling
2 Eggs benedict = 2900 kilojoules	2 eggs poached = 620 kilojoules	2280 kilojoules	Boiled eggs could also substitute, and save you a whole day's fat intake in one meal
Toasted muesli (½ cup) = 1030	Sultana Bran (1 cup) = 540 kilojoules	490 kilojoules	You get twice as much Sultana Bran and almost half the kilojoules compared to toasted muesli
Full-fat milk (250ml) = 675 kilojoules	Skim milk (250ml) = 365 kilojoules	310 kilojoules	Skim milk is by far and away the best choice over your cereal, or in smoothies

Day 60 tip – Move more

Use music to fire up your exercise routine

Just as you can use music to relax you or create a mood, music can add an exciting and fun element to exercise. People who listen to music while they exercise can experience a surprising range of benefits. One study showed that music listeners who ran and walked on a treadmill had greater endurance, worked out longer and felt better after the workout than those who exercised in silence. Another study showed that women pedalled 25% longer and men pedalled 30% longer on a stationary bike before feeling exhausted while listening to their favourite tunes. Music distracts you from the effort, so you are less likely to hold back, slow down or stop exercising. Music, especially with an upbeat tempo, can boost mood and happiness, and helps develop a more a positive attitude towards exertion.

Living it

Listening to music can motivate and distract you, making you exercise harder and longer. Just don't have it too loud if you're exercising near traffic.

Day 61 tip – Motivation and mindset

Accept responsibility for your weight

Only you can be responsible for what you think, how you feel and when you act. Maintaining your current level of body fat is a choice. To be blunt, you chose to stay fat. It may not feel like a choice, but you are choosing (by not doing anything) to reduce the quality and quantity of your life. You are in control, and you make the decision to change.

Living it

Only you can determine your priorities and goals. Don't waste your time blaming others for the choices, actions or inactions of the past. By all means, acknowledge any anger, hostility, pessimism, depression, past hurts, pains, abuse, mistreatment and misdirection, but look towards the future. There's always time to take charge and accept responsibility for your own behaviour thus determining the future direction of your life.

Day 62 tip – Good food

Don't blow out when you eat out

The ever-increasing reliance on foods eaten away from home isn't doing our waistlines any favours. Research has shown that the more often you eat out, the fatter you are likelier to become because food prepared away from home can contain up to 50% more kilojoules than a typical meal consumed at home. Most restaurant meals and takeaway foods have excess kilojoules because they are high in fat and large in portion size. Some fast-food meals can deliver your recommended daily kilojoules and fat intake in one meal.

Living it

Do your best to eat out less often; however, when you do here are some things you can do to minimise the damage.

- Look for lean meats and lots of vegetables

- Avoid anything battered, deep fried or covered in a cream sauce

- Only order a small glass of soft drink, fruit juice or alcohol, or drink water instead.

- If you order an entree or dessert, share it.

- Avoid feeling like you must clean your plate. You can usually take leftovers home

- Ask for salad dressings and sauces to be served on the side so you can have less.
- Avoid 'super size' or 'all you can eat' meals.

Day 63 tip – Move more

Measure your exercise intensity with perceived exertion

Another very helpful way to see if you are pushing yourself hard enough during exercise is the rate of perceived exertion (RPE) scale. This uses words on a scale of 0–10 to describe how hard you feel you are pushing yourself at the time. It's easy to use and is a fairly accurate guide to training at the right level to achieve your goals.

Living it

The following chart comes in many forms, but the one below is modified to help target weight and fat loss. As you can see, it's best to train at a somewhat strong level (rating 5) for optimal fat burning, although beginners should take it a little easier (rating 3–4) and you can go a little harder if you have been training for some time (rating 6–7). You can also spend short bursts of effort at the higher levels during interval training.

Rating	Exertion level	Type of conditioning
0	Complete rest	No movement/elite couch potato
1	Extremely easy	Incidental movement
2	Very easy	Warm up/cool down
3	Somewhat easy	Mild fat burning/beginner
4	Moderate	Moderate fat burning
5	Somewhat strong	Good fat burning
6	Hard	Advanced fat burning/mild fitness
7	Very hard	Some fat burning/fitness training
8	Very, very hard	Good fitness training
9	Extremely hard	Advanced fitness training
10	Maximal	Sprints/elite fitness training

Day 64 tip – Motivation and mindset

Determine your body fat percentage

Body fat percentage is an indication of the amount of fat on your body relative to your total body weight. It's useful for measuring your fat loss progress. Even if your actual body weight doesn't increase, the changing composition of your muscle/fat ratio can be encouraging. Until recently the only way to measure your body fat percentage was with skin fold calipers, but there are now easier methods of assessment.

Living it

In addition to special scales that you can purchase which send a harmless pulse through your body, you can now check your percentage of body fat with a simple calculation. The measure involves a standard formula for adjusting waist measurements by age and sex, and its accuracy is comparable to skin fold methods. The formulae and an example is shown below:

- **Males:** % body fat = (0.567 x waist in cm) + (0.0101 x age in years) – 31.8

- **Females:** % body fat = (0.439 x waist in cm) + (0.221 x age in years) – 9.4

- **Example:** A 24 year old female with a waist measurement of 78cm (0.439 x 78) + (0.221 x 24) – 9.4 = 30.146% body fat

---

Day 65 tip – Good food

Eat fat to lose fat (conditions apply)

Knowing the difference between good fats and bad fats is crucial for weight loss. There are some types of fats that actually help you to accelerate the removal, or prevent the storage of body fat. Dietary fats can either be used structurally (e.g. as an ingredient in hormones), for storage (in your fat cells) or metabolically (used for energy). Mono-unsaturated and polyunsaturated fats are much more likely to be used structurally and metabolically than saturated fats. The good fats are an important source of essential nutrients, which are the building blocks of hormones that help your body burn fat as fuel.

Living it

The fats found in seafood, lean meats, extra virgin olive oil, nuts, seeds and avocados are less likely to be stored as body fat, and provide essential nutrients that may actually help you lose weight. These fats are nutrient rich because they have minimal processing or chemical alteration, unlike the fats found in margarine, deep fried foods, doughnuts, biscuits and pastries. Moderate your portions of all fats, but try to get the majority of your fat intake from good fats.

Day 66 tip – Move more

Use sprintervals – and burn three times more fat in half the time

Interval training uses bursts of high intensity effort followed by recovery periods to dramatically boosts the kilojoule-burning, fat-burning and fitness-increasing benefits of exercise. Not only does it add variety, but look at what it can do to accelerate your results. A great study compared overweight women who cycled at a steady, constant state for 40 minutes with another group who cycled for 20 minutes, but performed frequent, intense 8 second bursts followed by a 12 second active rest. The interval group lost 3 times more weight. That's triple the weight loss in half the time. Training at a much higher level of intensity (in small tolerable doses) helps your body adapt to a higher level of fitness and stamina, especially if you have hit a plateau.

Living it

If there's one tip I can't stress enough, this is it. Unless you are a beginner, you should be doing intervals during your cardiovascular exercise to burn extra fat.

Day 67 tip – Motivation and mindset

Don't wait to feel motivated – do it now anyhow

Feeling motivated to exercise, and wanting to eat well can almost guarantee you success because you want to live the life that will ultimately get you results. There are no setbacks, no self-conflict, no point focusing on the foods you can't have. My hope is that this book gets you to that place, but realistically this type of motivation takes months to develop. Don't lay there idle waiting for it to magically appear. Getting started and staying on track when you're not motivated is the real challenge.

Living it

If you have been inactive for some time, I wouldn't expect you to feel motivated. But no matter how unmotivated you are, it's up to you to get started and get moving. No one else can do it for you. It could be as easy as a 10-minute walk. Then tomorrow, do it again. You probably won't feel motivated, and don't expect to be. Just get out there and do something. Begin the process, and gradually, the motivation will come. Over time, you'll find motivation in the doing. You will begin to feel better about yourself. When you start to have more energy and your clothes fit you better – that's motivating. Wellness is motivating, being unfit and overweight isn't. Don't wait till it's too late.

Day 68 tip – Good food

Choose a good breakfast cereal

There is a very diverse range of quality when it comes to breakfast cereals. Some cereals promoted for their weight-loss qualities rank among the worst choices after you look at the nutrition label, so it's important to sort through the hype. If your goal is to lose weight and fat, your cereal should be low in fat, salt and sugar, as well as high in quality carbohydrate and dietary fibre. This gives you maximum fullness and nutrition for minimum kilojoules. A recent study found that wholegrain cereals helped people lose weight while boosting their consumption of fibre, magnesium and vitamin B-6. This is important because it shows that you can cut kilojoules while maintaining or improving your nutrient intake.

Living it

Read the nutrition information panels, and look for:

Per 100g serving

Fat	5 grams or less
Sugar	10 grams or less
Fibre	4 grams or more
Sodium	250mg or less

Cereals that normally meet these criteria include wheat biscuits, natural muesli (although a little higher in fat), shredded wheat, oat or wheat bran and bran flakes. Add skim milk, fresh fruit and low-fat yoghurt.

Day 69 tip – Move more

Find a good training partner

A good training partner can be one of the best ways to stay motivated and make your exercise satisfying, stimulating and fun. It helps to have someone who depends on you, especially on those days when you don't feel like training. It's important to find a training partner with a shared focus on weight loss, especially someone who may even push you a little harder than you'd push yourself. Other qualities that make up a good training partner include:

- punctuality
- consistency
- honesty
- the ability to listen.

A training partner can also make it possible to participate in activities that you might not be able to undertake by yourself. For example, a training partner can play tennis with you, spot you at the gym or increase the safety of your evening walks.

Living it

Training partners are a bit like a personal trainer, where they help you stay motivated. By making a commitment to exercise with someone else, you're more likely to stick with it.

Day 70 tip – Motivation and mindset

Let's make this all about you

You are unique, so what works for your friend or partner may not work for you. Excess body fat is a symptom of many different problems and health considerations unique to each individual. You can't lose weight for your partner or your doctor – it's got to be about you. As an individual, you need to consider how important it is to apply lifestyle advice, and how to make it relevant to you. To achieve weight loss, you may need to put yourself first before other commitments. Once you realise that the very best parent, partner or employee you can be is a fit, energetic and happy one, it all becomes clear.

Living it

I acknowledge that some of the tips in this book may not be relevant to you or your lifestyle. So I encourage you to highlight the pages that are. Make note of the pages and tips that address something you really need to work on, or touch on an area that could have the greatest impact. You can then develop your own unique action plan to get results.

Day 71 tip – Good food

Learn how to crack the food label code (think 5–10)

Our supermarkets contain thousands of foods with all sorts of nutritional claims that can seem more complicated than the Da Vinci code. Learning how to decipher food labels can help you to make better food choices. Fat, sugar and salt is hidden in many foods, so it really helps to get an idea of exactly what you are eating.

Living it

Where possible, use the nutrition information tables, which must be included if a packaged food makes a health claim. Look for foods that are less than 5 grams of fat per 100 grams, and avoid foods that are over 10 grams of fat per 100 grams. This is the 5–10 rule, and it's a simple yet useful guide to fat content (except for high water content foods like milk or yoghurt). It's also beneficial to choose food with at least 3 grams of dietary fibre per 100 grams. Another aspect of food labels is their health claims. While some can be downright misleading, as you'll see later on day 86, others can be helpful, including those listed below.

Helpful claim	Translation
Low fat, low in fat	Must have no more than 3g of fat per 100g of food, or 1.5g of fat per 100ml of liquid food
Fat free	No more than 0.15g of fat per 100g
High fibre	This food has 3g of fibre or more per serving
Unsweetened	No added sugars and no artificial sweeteners
Diet	Contains at least 40% less kilojoules than the regular product; there must be a reduction of 170kj per 100g of food, or 80kj of liquids

Day 72 tip – Move more

Always strive to beat your best when exercising

Do you have a personal best walk, run, race time to beat or weight to lift? I can't stress enough the importance of having PBs (personal bests). Not only are PBs a great source of motivation, they are an essential ingredient to losing body fat, gaining strength and getting results. If you get obsessed with PBs (so that every weight you lift and every cardio workout you do, you want to beat your best) then you can't help but eventually get results. If you want to lose fat or get stronger, you'll need to continually compete against yourself. You'll need to work harder, faster, longer, or lift heavier weights if you want to achieve a personal best. Monitor your progress, time your activity, set yourself challenges and write down how much weight you lift. Beat your best consistently and you'll force your body to change.

Living it

Having a PB to beat is not only motivating, it's goal setting made simple. At least once or twice a week set a distance, time or lap challenge that fits in with your schedule, and try to improve on your previous best.

Day 73 tip – Motivation and mindset

Examine your beliefs, and your focus

Your beliefs and priorities help to form the foundation of a healthy lifestyle. They create a framework, or window, that helps to determine your mindset when making decisions and contemplating changes. Having a better understanding of yourself and why you want to succeed can help you to approach changes with confidence and determination. You have to genuinely believe that improving your health will add value back to all other aspects of your life. If not, you'll continue to put your work, social, spiritual and family life ahead of your health, and you'll struggle to take time away from these things to get serious results.

Living it

How strongly do you believe that you can make a change to your lifestyle and attitude? What are you prepared to give up? If you believe strongly that you can make changes, or acknowledge that you need to make changes, what can you do differently to get results? Could you cycle to work, catch up with friends for a walk instead of a meal, or have a picnic and kick a ball around with your family instead of going to the movies? Lifestyle changes have to become your focus, and not an inconvenient extra thing to do. Identify what stops you from improving your eating habits or activity levels? What aspects of your life could you modify to becoming healthier?

Day 74 tip – Good food

Know your ingredients

If a packaged food doesn't make a health claim, the only guide you have to its nutritional quality is the ingredients list. All packaged products must include a list of ingredients in order of quantity, where the first ingredient is the largest, and the last ingredient is the smallest (except water, which can always be listed last).

Living it

Cut back on foods that have fat or sugar listed in the first few ingredients, or that use different names for fat and sugar throughout the ingredients list. Some products use three or four different types of fats or sugars, which when added together would look a lot worse on a food label. Below is a table showing some of the different names for fats and sugars that you'll see on the ingredients list of food labels.

Different names for fat	Different names for sugar
Vegetable oil	Sucrose
Animal oil	Fructose
Shortening	Malt
Copha	Maltose
Lard	Lactose
Tallow	Glucose
Coconut oil	Treacle
Palm oil	Sorbitol
Butter fat	Mannitol
Milk solids	Invert sugar
Monoglycerides	Raw, brown and cane sugar
Chocolate or chocolate chips	Maple, golden and corn syrup

Day 75 tip – Move more

Lift weights to help you lose weight

Weight training, also known as resistance training, involves adding resistance to your body's natural movements to stimulate muscle strengthening. This resistance can be in the form of your body weight, a hand-held weight, pin-loaded weights, hydraulic resistance, elastic bands or water. Studies have shown that resistance training can help to decrease your body fat percentage and increase your muscle mass, resulting in a faster metabolic rate by around 7–8%.

Living it

Don't be daunted by this wonderful form of exercise. Aim to do 2 days a week in addition to your cardiovascular exercise, and make sure you have at least one rest day in between lifting weights. Try to minimise your rest between sets and between exercises to maximise kilojoule burning. You'll find more guidelines on strength training throughout this book.

Day 76 tip – Motivation and mindset

Work from the inside out, not the outside in

The most important aspect to changing your lifestyle is your desire to take action. There's no point forcing changes upon yourself that you don't really want to make because you won't stick with it. Your lifestyle changes have to be in harmony with the true person that you are. Weight-loss tips are helpful, but all the knowledge in the world won't make any difference unless you want to act on it.

Living it

Don't try and lose weight to make yourself a happier person. Work on being a happier person first, such as dealing with stress, prioritising yourself, setting goals, rewarding yourself and addressing any issues that relate to overeating. You'll then be in a far better place to challenge the behaviours and habits that are preventing you from losing weight.

Day 77 tip – Good food

Eat more beans, peas and lentils (legumes)

If the only legumes you've ever eaten are baked beans and a little humus dip, it's time to step out of your comfort zone. Legumes (sometimes called pulses) are pretty much the ideal fat loss food, giving you maximum fullness for minimum kilojoules. They are high in protein and fibre, and low in fat, which makes them good at regulating your blood sugar and insulin levels and making you feel full. They come canned in many varieties, so you can use them immediately without soaking. Here are some ideas on how you could include more legumes in your diet:

- Lentils, black-eyed peas and split peas are great in soups
- Use pinto or refried beans in burritos
- Add red lentils to a curry, stew or casserole
- Use red kidney beans in chili con carne
- Add white cannellini beans or chickpeas to a minted salad.

Living it

Look for ways to include legumes in your diet at least two or three times a week. Along with water-rich vegetables, they are the ideal food for weight loss.

Day 78 tip – Move more

Don't worry about your muscles bulking up if you lift weights

Let me make this clear – you will not get bulky from lifting weights. This is the most unfortunate health and fitness myth of all because it discourages people from lifting weights and they miss out on some wonderful, weight reducing benefits. Very few men and even fewer women have the genetic potential to build bulky muscles. Even if they do, it requires near full-time dedication to a lifestyle that demands very heavy lifting, adequate sleep, a strict high-protein diet, supplementation and, in some cases, injections of various substances.

Living it
The type of resistance training I encourage involves manageable weights and higher repetition ranges, helping you to become strong, firm, energised and healthy looking. You will not get big. Let's mark this myth as 'busted'.

Day 79 tip – Motivation and mindset
Keep your expectations realistic
If you expect fast results, you can expect fast frustration. Slow and steady weight loss may not sound exciting but it's the only way that works over the long-term. I acknowledge that it's difficult to stick with lifestyle changes when you don't get results as fast as you expect. But it's often your expectations that are the root of your frustration. You need to make slow, gradual changes and expect slow, gradual results. The benefits from exercise and healthy eating come in weeks and months, not in minutes. If you approach weight and fat loss realistically, you'll be much more likely to succeed.

Living it
It helps to be clear about what to expect and when to expect it. Keep the following in mind:

- Expect lifestyle changes to be challenging (but achievable)
- Expect weight and fat loss to be slow
- Expect to see plateaus in your results (you can't lose weight continuously)
- Expect the changes you make to your diet to be long-term
- Expect there to be setbacks along the way.

Day 80 tip – Good food
Don't eat in front of the television
One of the main reasons that TV viewing increases your chances of being overweight is because of what it does to your eating behaviour. One study found that for each hour of TV viewing, subjects ate an additional 700 kilojoules (167 calories) on top of their daily kilojoule intake. Another study showed that children ate 20–25% of their daily kilojoules while watching TV, especially on weekends. Eating in front of the TV can have a negative impact on your weight in three ways:

- You are more likely to snack and nibble while watching TV (and less likely to be active)
- You are more likely to eat junk in front of the TV, possibly because of the influence of TV advertising
- You may eat larger portions as you are distracted to the extent that internal fullness signals from the stomach go unnoticed.

Living it

Try not to snack or eat while you watch TV, especially something out of a packet where you have no idea what your portion size is. If you must snack, make sure it is a healthy choice, and even so, dish yourself up a small portion before you sit down in front of the box to prevent distracted eating.

Day 81 tip – Move more

Keep an exercise journal

An exercise journal helps to monitor your exercise habits and keep you on track. Unlike a food diary, an exercise journal can be a more permanent addition to your routine because it keeps a record of your progress. It's hard to progress if you just turn up at the gym and mindlessly hop on an exercise machine. A well-kept exercise journal can tell you how fast, how far, for how long you went last time, so you have a measure to improve upon. The same applies to lifting weights

Living it

Writing things down is a genuine commitment to change and to getting results. Record details like the type of exercise you are doing, how long you are doing it for, and how far you have travelled. Walkers can use a pedometer to keep track of their steps, kilojoules burned and distance travelled. It should only take you a few seconds each day to note down all your details. You can also review your journal over time and see how far you have come.

Day 82 tip – Motivation and mindset

Face the impact of the number 82

What is so significant about the number 82, According to the Australian Institute of Health and Welfare, 82 is the average life expectancy of Australian men and women. While it does differ over different age groups and genders, this is a fairly accurate figure to go by.

Living it

Subtract your age from 82, and have a long, hard look at that number. According to a range of forecasts and averages, that's how long you have left to make a difference to your quality and quantity of life. This is not meant to depress you but rather to make you see that life is too short to feel tired, unwell and unhealthy. When you don't have all that long and you know what you want, what are you waiting for?

Day 83 tip – Good food

Make your breakfast healthy, even when you're in a rush

Are you more likely to grab some fast food for breakfast when you're busy or rushed? With a little planning, a fast morning meal can take little or no time to prepare and minimal time to consume. Try these ideas for a fast and healthy breakfast:

- If you have no time, choose foods such as yoghurt, low-fat muesli bars or a commercial breakfast drink that can be consumed on the go
- Choose fruit that you can eat easily on the run, such as bananas, apples, strawberries, pears, peaches, grapes and mandarins
- Traditional breakfast foods such as fruit, wholegrain cereal (with skim milk) or toast (minimal butter or margarine) are very easy to prepare and provide fibre with very little fat
- Prepare the ingredients for a fruit smoothie and refrigerate before you go to bed.

Living it

No matter how frantic things are for you in the morning, there are healthy choices available that take little or no time to prepare.

Day 84 tip – Move more

Include activities that you enjoy

If you can include activities in your exercise routine that you really enjoy, you'll be much more likely to stick to it. You will feel enthusiastic and look forward to the activity rather than making excuses to avoid it. As exercise becomes more of a habit, you'll start to feel fitter and more energetic. You might even feel bad if you miss a day of exercise. Eventually, you might find yourself wanting to be active on your weekends or on holidays instead of lazing around doing nothing. Suddenly, one of your friends might call you a fitness freak.

Living it

Is there an activity you have always wanted to try, or something that you once enjoyed and would like to get back into? Experiment with a wide variety of activities to increase your chances of finding something that's right for you. By finding an activity you are passionate about, exercise will never seem like a chore. When you try some new activities or do them at a different intensity, keep an open mind and ease into them. You can even include some activities that are more about fun than exercise, such as table tennis, backyard cricket, throwing a frisbee or flying a kite with your kids.

Day 85 tip – Motivation and mindset

Aim for improvement, not perfection

A mild degree of perfectionism can encourage you to strive towards being your best, and give you the motivation to persevere under adversity. But aiming for the perfect diet or the perfect body is a recipe for failure because they are near impossible to attain. This can result in feelings of frustration, stress, anxiety, sadness and guilt. It can also result in procrastination and inaction because perfectionists become reluctant to start a new task, fearing they may fail.

Living it

Perfection is a difficult trait to overcome, but you can step back from the need to be perfect by trying to:

- set a realistic and flexible time frame for weight loss
- reward yourself for progress, not completion
- not criticise or expect perfection in others
- expect setbacks and failings, and forgive yourself
- indulge occasionally then get straight back on track.

Day 86 tip – Good food

Don't fall for the food label traps

A lot of the nutrition claims you see on food labels can be confusing at best and bordering on misleading at worst.

Living it

Here are some of the more confusing label claims and what they actually mean.

Confusing claim	Translation
Lite or light	May have no relation to fat content. It could relate to flavour or salt, or even colour in the case of 'light' oil. Look for the characteristic that makes the food light.
Contains real fruit, or contains real fruit pulp	Food manufacturers must show the actual percentage of real fruit in the ingredients list, so make sure you look. One product that 'contains real fruit' has just 0.2% fruit juice. It's pretty hard to justify the claim on the label, but legally they can do it.
Reduced, less and lower fat	This does not mean low fat, although it is has at least 25% less fat than regular foods in the same category. Also, it must be 3g per 100g less than the regular food.
% fat free	This is the most confusing. For example, 90% fat free is still very high in fat. The fat percentage is listed by weight.
No cholesterol, cholesterol free	This does not mean low fat. Plant foods like peanut butter, coconut cream or avocados can't contain cholesterol, but you'll still see the cholesterol free claims. Saturated fat must be below 20% of the total fat content, while unsaturated fat must be above 40%.
All natural	Refers to a food with only natural food additives and flavours. For example, tinned fruit in fruit juice. It's virtually meaningless.
No added sugar	No added sugar (sucrose), honey, malt, glucose syrup or fruit juice, but these claims are most often found on products fairly high in natural sugars, such as fruit juice and jam.

Day 87 tip – Move more

Do cardio instead of sit-ups to lose fat off your tummy

There is no doubt that sit-ups with controlled, correct technique can strengthen your abdominals. But they do nothing to get rid of the fat sitting over the top of the muscle. Want proof? A group of people performed sit-ups every day for a month, and they lost no more fat off their stomachs than they did off their unexercised buttocks or upper back. You can't spot reduce or choose where the fat comes off you. Chewing gum all day won't rid you of a double chin. That's up to your own unique balance of hormone. You are better off spending 5–10 minutes going for a jog, or doing a few sprints to ramp up your metabolism. The key to losing fat off your stomach (in order of preference) is:

1. Healthy, tasty, long-term, low-kilojoule eating
2. Combining that with regular cardiovascular exercise and interval training
3. Boosting your metabolism with adequate sleep and functional strength training.

Living it

To lose fat off your tummy, or any part of your body, don't worry about sit-ups. They say that abs are made in the kitchen, so don't neglect your healthy eating. In addition, aerobic exercises such as walking and running are the best investment of your time.

Day 88 tip – Motivation and mindset

Look to the long-term. It'll help you in the short-term

A recent study discovered that one of the major determinants of success was a mindset with a long time perspective. People who took the future into consideration with every current decision they had to make were more likely to succeed. On the other hand, the hope of instant gratification, such as the tendency to want instant dieting success, is a primary cause of failure.

Living it

Taking a long-term view of your pursuit of better health is one of the most important single factors determining your long-term success. It's one of the reasons that fad diets don't work because you know deep inside you'll never stick to it. Look at everything you do in terms of its long-term potential impact on your health. Take time to make small changes, and realise that what seems like a small sacrifice now (cooking instead of buying takeaway, or exercising instead of watching TV) will ultimately lead to greater results in the future.

Day 89 tip – Good food

Become less refined and use fewer white carbs

The type of carbohydrates you eat can have just as much influence over your body shape as the amount. Research has shown that people who are overweight do not appear to eat more carbohydrates overall than people who weigh less. However, overweight people tend to eat more refined carbohydrates, such as white bread, rice and pasta, which cause a rapid increase in blood sugar. Refined carbohydrates are also found in processed foods that contain a lot of sugar. The body stores easily digested carbohydrates in your muscles and liver, but if there's too much, or if you don't burn it off through exercise, it can be converted into body fat. Too much refined carbohydrates can also make it harder to burn off the fat in your diet because your body tends to burn off carbohydrates first.

Living it

Cut back or cut out on highly processed carbohydrate foods such as white bread, white rice, white pasta and low-fibre breakfast cereals. You'll need bigger servings of these foods to feel full, and they have a negative impact on your blood sugar levels. Choose the wholegrain varieties instead.

Day 90 tip – Move more

Use hills, stairs or sand to up the intensity of your walks

Do you hate the hills, or power up them? Walking is a great fat-burning exercise, but once you get to a reasonable level of fitness, you have to go further, faster and more often to maintain its effectiveness. If you stay at the same pace, you'll actually start to burn fewer kilojoules because you may weigh a little less, or your body may have become more efficient. The nature of the surface you walk on has a strong influence on the amount of kilojoules you burn. Walking in the sand will cushion any impact, and it also burns more kilojoules because the 'give' when your foot pushes down forces your body and muscles to work harder to keep you moving. Hills and stairs also offer the same benefits and intensity of running without any impact.

Living it

When you're out and about walking, look for hills and stairs to add extra intensity. If you live near the beach, schedule regular walks on the sand for added cushioning, variation and intensity.

Day 91 tip – Motivation and mindset

If you build on it, they will come (results that is)

Fat and weight loss is a slow journey and you need to make long-term changes to your lifestyle to achieve long-term results. Think of it like building a pyramid; the more solid and stable your foundations, the higher and more stable your eventual success will be. Gradually introduce manageable lifestyle changes, after you have others set in stone. Over time the small changes stack up, helping you to gain real, long-term results. This also keeps you motivated, helping to avoid the return of old habits that weren't working for you.

Living it

Start with a few small, easy to manage changes to your lifestyle; choose from the many in this book, but don't do too many at once. This is a better approach than throwing yourself in too deep and dramatically changing your whole life in one go. Remember, the tortoise won the race.

Day 92 tip – Good food

Watch what you eat with alcohol

Not only can alcohol put the brakes on your weight loss, so can the foods usually consumed with it. Some typical waist expanding combinations include beer and pizza, beer and hot dogs, beer and hot chips (at sporting events), wine with cheese and dips, and beer with nuts or crisps. Because alcohol is the type of fuel your body uses first, it makes it harder for your body to burn off all the kilojoules from these high-fat foods. So it's not necessarily a beer gut, but a beer and chips gut. It's also important to realise that when alcohol is consumed during a meal, the extra kilojoules are not normally compensated for by eating less food. So you end up with a higher than normal kilojoule intake and a bigger mountain to climb to achieve weight and fat loss.

Living it

Many people enjoy crunchy, salty foods while they have an alcoholic beverage. Following are some tasty food choices that can have less of an impact on your waistline. (It's also good to have water between drinks.)

- pretzels
- coloured rice crackers
- rice cracker biscuits with tomato salsa
- rice cracker biscuits with humus
- rice cracker biscuits with bean dips
- blanched vegetable sticks with dips
- salted fat-free popcorn
- crunchy bread sticks.

Day 93 tip – Move more

Exercise when you're hungry, especially before breakfast

When you first wake up in the morning, your blood sugar levels are generally low because you haven't eaten for several hours while your metabolism has been burning off kilojoules. This creates a unique opportunity, where your low blood sugar levels force your body to tap into stored fat to provide fuel for your exercise. You don't necessarily burn more kilojoules in total, but you burn off a higher proportion of fat as fuel than you would if you did an identical workout after breakfast. Research shows that before breakfast up to 50% more fat is used during cardiovascular exercise compared to people doing an identical amount of exercise after breakfast. There is an argument that exercise on an empty stomach will be less intense and therefore less effective because you are low in energy. But, this is really only a concern to diabetics and elite athletes.

Living it

Try exercising first thing in the morning on an empty stomach. Water or black, sugarless coffee is okay beforehand. Even if you do this just a few days a week, it can help to make your exercise more effective.

Day 94 tip – Motivation and mindset

Manage your time to manage your weight

Because a healthier lifestyle is important but not urgent, any pressing issues can often jump to the top of your priority list. When you've already got too much to do, and too little time, finding the time to exercise or prepare healthy meals can be a challenge. Feeling overwhelmed can lead to stress, unhappiness and loss of control. So why not try a little time management?

It's not about squeezing more tasks and activities into your day, but rather a way of helping you focus on getting the important things done and using your time more effectively.

Living it

Use the tips below to help save you precious minutes every day, giving you extra time to look after your health.

- When faced with a new email or piece of paper, apply the FAT principle (File, Act or Toss).

- Imagine the difference it would make if you could double your reading and typing speed.

- Cut back on the amount of TV you watch, or use your TV viewing time wisely. Do some weights or stretches, or make lunch for the next day.

- Set priorities, make a to-do list and allocate your time towards the most valuable, rewarding tasks.

- Work smarter, not harder. Identify when your most productive hours of the day are and use that time to focus on your top priorities.

- Screen your calls to prevent interruptions. Important callers will get back to you, or leave a message, and you can stay focused on the task at hand.

Day 95 tip – Good food

Enjoy a lean and luscious lunch to maximise energy and weight loss

A healthy lunch can boost your energy levels and prevent you from feeling sluggish throughout the afternoon. It doesn't need to be a huge meal, otherwise you might end up feeling like an afternoon siesta. Skipping lunch will not accelerate weight loss, and can actually make things worse by making you crave junk food.

Living it

Try to be organised for your lunch to prevent any reliance on fast food. Aim for a quality wholegrain type food, a low-fat protein-based food, and some fibrous vegetables. If you don't have time to make your own healthy lunch, here are some better choices when you're on the run:

- fresh sushi
- salads with low-fat dressings
- lean meat and wholegrain bread salad sandwiches

- wraps with lean meats and salad vegetables
- vegetable and chicken soup with a crusty, wholegrain roll.

Day 96 tip – Move more

Push yourself hard enough to hear your breath during cardiovascular exercise

Can you hear yourself puff when you exercise? One of the main problems with activities like walking and cycling on a stationary bike is that it's too easy to take it easy. If you want to make sure your exercise is burning fat, and that you are pushing yourself hard enough, your breath can actually be a very helpful and easy-to-use guide. A recent study showed that when you start to hear your breath during exercise, you're working at about 60–65% of your maximum heart rate. This is a good level of exertion for burning fat.

Living it

When you exercise, try to push yourself to a level where you are puffing and can hear your own breath. You don't have to be gasping or uncomfortable. As you get fitter, this will still be a helpful guide, as you'll have to push yourself a little harder to make yourself puff.

Day 97 tip – Motivation and mindset

Focus on the process, not the results

Instead of obsessing about your weight or girth measurements, try to focus your attention on the process of improving your lifestyle. These are the little things you do every day and every week, like healthier eating and regular exercise. Focusing on your results (your weight) can be counter-productive because you set yourself up for disillusionment. It's an emotional roller-coaster ride that can be very de-motivating when you don't achieve what you expect. This is even more frustrating when you focus on weight, which can fluctuate by up to 2 kilograms a day due to changes in your fluid levels. You can't control your results, but you can control what you do to get results. Focus on the results, and the process may get frustrating; focus on the process, and the results will come.

Living it

Judge your progress by your behaviour and tasks completed, not your weight. That's how you get results, not by weighing yourself every day. This is particularly important for people who have had a history of failure on weight-loss programs. Some helpful process measures are given in the table following.

Healthy eating	Physical activity
Daily water-rich vegetable intake (4 serves) Breakfast eaten daily Daily fat intake Daily water intake Reduced junk food intake Days without alcohol Lower portion sizes	Daily steps taken Number of days of activity in a week Distance covered during exercise Total minutes exercised Not missing 2 days in a row Reduced car usage Heart rate measurements

Day 98 tip – Good food

Five simple lunch swaps to make those kilos drop

If you can find dietary changes that sacrifice kilojoules without sacrificing taste, you are on a sure fire winner.

Living it

Here are five small things you can do at lunch to make a big difference to your results over time.

Instead of...	Go for...	Save...	Comments
Mayonnaise (1 tbsp) = 310 kilojoules	Chutney (1 tbsp) = 145 kilojoules	165 kilojoules	Low-fat mayonnaise has the same kilojoule content as chutney
Caesar salad = 1850 kilojoules	Thai beef salad = 415 kilojoules	1435 kilojoules	Make a healthy caesar salad for yourself, or ask for the sauce on the side
Vegetarian foccacia = 2700 kilojoules	Sushi (6 pieces) = 820 kilojoules	1880 kilojoules	Sushi is much lower in kilojoules and fat; go for salmon to get those good fats
Cream chicken soup (1 cup) = 550 kilojoules	Vegetable soup (1 cup) = 235 kilojoules	315 kilojoules	With half the kilojoules, and triple the fibre content, vegetable soup is a tasty swap
Flat bread = 470 kilojoules	2 lettuce leaves = 10 kilojoules	460 kilojoules	For your wrap, use iceberg lettuce instead of flat bread; it's like a cold san choy bow

---

Day 99 tip – Move more

Wait as long as you can to eat after exercise (for fat loss)

Do you feel hot, sweaty and red faced after your workout? If you do, that's great because you've boosted your metabolic rate. Your body is burning stored fat and kilojoules at a higher rate than normal, which is a vital step in changing your body shape. But as soon as you eat something, the glucose that enters your blood stream will become the first choice of fuel to be used instead of stored fuel. So to maximise the use of stored fat as fuel, try to avoid eating for 30–45 minutes after working out. Just be aware that this strategy is not recommended for diabetics.

It's also the opposite of what you would do if your exercise goal was to get aerobically fit, where you would eat or drink a high glycemic food as soon as possible to replenish glycogen stores.

Living it

After exercise, only drink water, and wait as long as you can before eating. When you do eat, make it a high-protein, moderate carbohydrate and low-fat food, such as low-fat yoghurt, a high-fibre cereal with skim milk, or a fruit smoothie.

Day 100 tip – Motivation and mindset

Make sure you don't suffer from couch potato contentment

A recent survey revealed that many overweight and obese people were completely or somewhat satisfied with their physical health. This seems to indicate a serious level of misunderstanding about the dangers of excess body fat. Don't let your expanding waistline become the norm. Just because they are now making airline seats bigger to accommodate our ever-expanding girths, you don't have to feel obliged to fill in the space.

Living it

While it may seem easier to stay fat than to do something about it, there are serious health issues to consider. Following are some important reasons why you shouldn't get too comfortable when there is a bulge over your belt.

- Obesity is worse for your health than a lifetime smoking habit, or chronic drinking.
- If your waist measurement is over 101cm (for men) or over 91cm (for women), body fat is placing your health at risk right now.

- Obesity has been shown to reduce your lifespan by up to 20 years.
- Excess body fat significantly increases your chances of developing type 2 diabetes.
- Excess weight stresses our internal organs, puts pressure on joints and can interfere with our posture and gait, thereby messing with the spine.

Day 101 tip – Good food

Switch to skim milk, and leave the full-fat milk for the calves

It's easy to be confused about the percentage of fat in full-cream milk. By weight, full-cream milk is only 4% fat. This seems amazing, and the dairy industry actually promoted this heavily a few years back. But a lot of the weight of milk is water. If you measure the fat content by kilojoules, full-cream milk is actually more than 50% fat. The most practical thing to look at is how much fat you get per serving. A regular serving of milk is usually 1 cup or 250ml, which is about what you'd pour over a bowl of cereal. A regular serving of full-cream milk provides 10 grams of fat, while the same amount of skim milk contains 0.3 grams of fat. By making this simple change, you'll consume about 3 kilograms less saturated animal fat each year. Also confusing was the recent study that showed women who consumed whole milk gained less weight over time. But the finer details showed that this was only relevant to women who were of normal weight at the start of the study. It wasn't for weight loss. The study also failed to look at other habits that aided their weight control.

Living it

If you drink a lot of milk (e.g. on breakfast cereal or in a smoothie), skim milk is by far and away your best option. If you only have one or two teaspoons of milk in your tea or coffee, and you don't drink more than two cups a day, it hardly matters what milk you choose.

Day 102 tip – Move more

Use cross-training to boost your results, and motivation

Do you get bored doing the same type of exercise all the time? Cross-training is where you alternate a number of different activities in your exercise program. Using a wider variety of exercises can really help you to stay motivated, keeping your mind and body fresh. It can also help you to lose weight and fat, as long as you continue to focus on fat-burning activities. It will also reduce your risk of injury from one activity that continually stresses the same muscles and joints. Cross-training allows some muscle groups to rest while you train others, and gives you the training advantages of a broad range of activities.

Living it

If your primary focus is fat loss, intersperse activities like brisk walking, sand walking, jogging, cycling, aquarobics, paddling, gym classes and exercise equipment. You could also consider strength training or team sports depending on how much fat you have to lose.

Day 103 tip – Motivation and mindset

Work on your attitude. You are what you think

They say your attitude determines your altitude. With that in mind, you'll find it pretty hard to get great results with a negative attitude. Research shows that pessimists often neglect their health because they don't feel they will be successful at changing it. Negative thought patterns can fester in all aspects of our lives. For example, if one or two annoying things happen in the morning, we tell ourselves that it's going to be a bad day. We then spend the rest of the day focusing on what's gone wrong. Just as there are bad food habits, you can have bad thinking habits. The way you think can make a big difference, and there's no reason why you can't change your thought processes. If you have negative thoughts, dispute them. Be aware of your thoughts, and what you think to yourself. Optimists see change as a challenge. Are there any changes you could make to your attitude?

Living it

A big part of your success will depend on your attitude. Try to have a positive outlook towards all the changes and challenges you'll face. For example, you may not love exercise but it will help you get results, so why not make the most of it. Look for ways to make it more enjoyable, such as exercising to music because you'll be much more likely to stick with it.

Day 104 tip – Good food

Get your five servings of vegetables a day

Eating five servings of vegetables a day will do wonders for your weight and general health. But that doesn't mean you should eat five carrots a day.

Living it

Below are some helpful guidelines on how to choose vegetables.

- **Select one rich in vitamin A** – Good examples are carrots, spinach, sweet potato, winter squashes, broccoli and most dark green leafy vegetables.

- **Select one rich in vitamin C** – Examples are red capsicum, red chili, tomatoes and broccoli.

- **Select one high in fibre** – These include corn, squash, artichokes, parsnips, leafy greens, broccoli and cauliflower. Wash vegetables such as carrots and potatoes instead of peeling them to maximise fibre.

- **Select one from the cruciferous family** – These are plants bearing cross-shaped flowers, including cabbage, broccoli, brussels sprouts, cauliflower, kale, collards, mustard greens and turnips.

- **Select one based on colour** – Different colours provide different nutrients, so try to have something red, green, orange, yellow and white. A rainbow of colour adds to the visual appeal of your food.

Day 105 tip – Move more

When you start out at weight training, less is more

It's long been conventional strength training wisdom that you need to perform two or even three sets of repetitions of each exercise to maximise results. However, a recent study has debunked this theory, at least for beginners. Two groups lifted weights three times a week for 14 weeks; one group performed one set of each exercise, and another group performed three sets. The two groups increased strength and muscle density at virtually identical rates, which translates into less time lifting weights for the same results.

Living it

This is great for fat loss because you can still achieve modest gains in strength and muscle tone in less time. That's time you could invest in fat-burning cardiovascular exercise. Just don't forget the importance of a cardiovascular warm-up should you choose to do just one set. Other studies have shown that one-set training is mostly beneficial to beginners, so you may need to add an additional set after about 3–4 months.

Day 106 tip – Motivation and mindset

Start a small winning streak

If you think consistency is boring, why not try some public streaking? Being consistent with your exercise, healthy eating and attitude adjustments will no doubt help you get results, but you can also use it to help you stay motivated. Sticking to the food and exercise changes you have made is like starting a winning streak of success. Keeping that streak going, even for a short time, is a real motivator, helping to breed confidence and positivity. You might even get a rush out of keeping the streak alive for as long as you can. Starting a food or exercise related streak can also rub off on other parts of your life, like improving your sleep habits or managing your stress. Winning streaks are contagious.

Living it

Begin with a small change that will improve your chances of weight loss, like switching to skim milk. Stick to it for a week and you'll feel like you've made a good start. Stick to it for 2 weeks and you've really achieved something. Stick to it for 3 weeks and your taste buds start to adjust, and you'll find you don't miss full-cream milk quite so much. Stick to it for another week, and you'll have a new level of confidence when you make another change, like including a few more hills in your morning walks. You've started a winning streak, and keeping that streak alive has helped you unleash the power of consistency. Set a timeline to make your streaks more motivating, even if it's a weekly or fortnightly challenge. Others might prefer to exercise every day for a month, or drink 6 glasses of water every day for 60 days. Keep it fun, and don't worry if you break your streak. Just try to beat it next time. There are hundreds of examples of small lifestyle changes you could make throughout *Lighten Up*. What will you do to start your own winning streak?

Day 107 tip – Good food

Use protein to help you lose body fat, but don't get obsessed

Protein has a very significant role in helping you lose weight. Protein-rich foods help to satisfy your appetite, maintain your muscle mass after lowering your kilojoule intake, and boost your metabolic rate. Research has shown that lower kilojoule diets that have a higher proportion of protein and less from carbohydrates can accelerate fat loss faster than high-carbohydrate, lower protein diets of an equal kilojoule content. Studies have also shown that lower carbohydrate/high-protein diets were twice as good at maintaining the body's metabolic rate, and also promoted greater feelings of fullness from an equivalent amount of food. Protein is not a magical food, so don't go for too much of a good thing, but it will help the process of fat loss.

Living it

Choose your protein-rich foods wisely, as they often come loaded with fat. Look for lean meats, seafood, pulses, low-fat dairy products, eggs (go easy on the yolks) and moderate portions of nuts. It's also important to eat lean protein in combination with an increase in high fibre foods such as vegetables, fruits, whole grains and pulses. This helps to maintain a high fibre and high nutrient intake, and avoids some of the dangers associated with higher protein intake.

Day 108 tip – Move more

Trade off your indulgences

So you've had your indulgence, or you know one is coming up. That can't be changed, but you can trade off your indulgences and reduce the impact on your weight.

Living it

Here are three strategies you can use to regain some balance after indulging. A combination of all methods will prove to be most successful.

- **Do extra exercise** – When you do indulge, exchange it for some extra exercise and movement above and beyond your normal amount of exercise. For example, you could walk an extra 10 minutes for every standard alcoholic drink you consumed. It doesn't matter if you do your exercise the day before, the day of, or the day after your indulgence, but try to do something to make up for it.

- **Eat really well** – Try to only drink water, and eat a very low-kilojoule meal before and after your indulgence. You could try a vegetable stir-fry or tuna salad.

- **Learn for next time** – Plan for occasions where you have experienced social pressures or limited food choices in the past. Eat healthy foods before you go, take healthy foods with you or eat smaller portions. You can also learn which trading off strategies work best for you.

Day 109 tip – Motivation and mindset

Have a plan – be prepared for getting in shape

Weight loss is just like any other aspect of your life in that the more planning and preparation you do, the more likely you are to succeed. Preparation is a forgotten friend when it comes to weight loss. You don't have to be obsessive; but planning, organisation and structure can produce great results. It's a way to create and support change, and extra support can help you achieve amazing things in a relatively short period of time. People who plan ahead are more likely to see patterns in their behaviour, stay focused for longer, are less likely to make bad decisions, and consistently produce better results than people who aren't organised.

Living it

Think about what actions you need to take to get results. Don't leave decisions about what to eat to the last minute. Write down your planned meals for the week, including the meals you'll have on what nights. Add the necessary ingredients to your shopping list. Try to include recipes that you can make a double batch of, and freeze the leftovers for those nights when you know you'll be tired, or home late. Think about what exercise you are going to do this week, what days are best, and get your training gear ready before you go to bed. Make appointments with yourself in your diary, and plot your course.

Day 110 tip – Good food

Use powders if you struggle to eat enough protein

As we know, protein is important for fat loss because it helps you lose mostly fat and not muscle when you lower your kilojoule intake, keeping your metabolism running in high gear. On the other hand, too much protein can be dangerous for your health. The following table helps to calculate your exact daily protein needs. Multiply your weight by the relevant factor to see how many grams of protein you need every day. You can see that someone who is cutting back on their kilojoule intake needs close to 50% more protein compared to someone who is inactive.

Activity or other factor	Grams of protein per kilo of body weight
Sedentary adult	0.85
Recreational exerciser, adult	1.1–1.6
Adult restricting kilojoules	1.3–1.5 (a little more for men)

Living it

Many people are surprised at how much protein they should be eating to help with weight loss. Start at the low end of the scale, especially if you have a small frame, or are over 90 kilograms. Below is a list of the amount of protein in some common foods. If you struggle to get enough through diet, try some of the whey or soy-based protein powders that you can add to skim milk or water to help boost your intake.

Food	Grams of protein per serving (approx.)
Baked beans (½ cup)	8
Cottage cheese (½ cup)	15
Egg (1)	6
Fish, beef, chicken (90 grams)	20
Milk (1 cup – all types)	8
Nuts (¼ cup)	6
Protein powder (1 scoop)	20

Day 111 tip – Move more

Embrace the burn, but stop if you feel pain

Exercise shouldn't be too easy, but it also shouldn't be too hard. I like to make a clear distinction between a burn and pain. A burn is a feeling in your muscles or lungs when you are exercising reasonably hard, but within your capabilities. It gives you an awareness of your movement in a place where you would expect it to be based on the exercise you are doing. You also may feel like you can continue with the activity a little longer at the same intensity. On the other hand, pain in your joints, neck, back or elsewhere that limits your movement and feels uncomfortable should be seen as a warning sign. You should stop what you are doing, and not work through the pain.

Living it

A gentle burn during exercise is to be encouraged, but if you experience pain or suffer any of the following symptoms, stop immediately and see your doctor.

- chest pain/tightness
- severe breathlessness

- heart palpitations
- dizziness or light headedness.

Day 112 tip – Motivation and mindset

Progress through the stages of change

Making the change to a healthier lifestyle doesn't occur as a single event but through a series of identifiable stages.

Living it

Look at the stages of change below to see where you fit. We all go through these stages when making decisions to change our habits, and awareness can then help you to seek out what type of information or services you need to accelerate your journey through each stage. Finding ways to stay longer in the action and maintenance stages with fewer episodes in the relapse stage will be vital to your long-term success.

- **Pre-contemplation** – This could also be called denial, where you are unaware of, or doubt the benefits of making lifestyle changes. You are pessimistic about your ability to change, and do not intend to change anytime soon.

- **Contemplation** – You are considering change by weighing up the costs, effort, treatment and time commitment of a healthier lifestyle, although you may remain in this stage for months or even years.

- **Preparation** – You've decided to do something. You have made a time, set a date and found a course of action that you are comfortable with.

- **Action** – You are doing it. Your behaviour and habits are starting to change. You are walking regularly, planning meals and/or keeping a food diary. Be wary of falling back into the contemplation phase.

- **Maintenance** – This is the most desirable phase to be in. You are living it and loving it, and have successfully maintained a healthier lifestyle for more than 3–6 months.

- **Relapse** – Falling back to your old habits and abandoning your new behaviour. This is one we hope to avoid with a long-term approach.

Day 113 tip – Good food

Drink water before your meals to reduce hunger

Here's a great way to 'trick' your body into eating less kilojoules without feeling hungry. It's based on the fact that the amount of food you eat is linked to how full you feel. By drinking water 10 minutes before eating, you'll reduce the amount of kilojoules you eat afterwards. The chart below shows how many kilojoules subjects ate after drinking different volumes of water roughly 10 minutes before eating lunch. The results show that the larger the volume of water consumed before lunch, the fewer kilojoules were consumed at lunch.

Volume of water	Kilojoules eaten after water
No water	4334 kilojoules (1032 calories)
300 millilitres	3184 kilojoules (758 calories)
450 millilitres	2932 kilojoules (698 calories)
600 millilitres	2625 kilojoules (625 calories)

Living it

It's not just about drinking water but when you drink your water that can make a difference to your weight. Drinking water before a meal helps signal to the brain that you are full sooner, and you eat fewer kilojoules. Use this to your advantage by drinking at least 600 millilitres of water (the size of a typical bottle) around 10 minutes before you have lunch and dinner.

Day 114 tip – Move more

Use a pedometer, and aim for 10,000 steps each day

It seems like everyone these days has a pedometer, and with good reason. They are cheap and they help you track your exercise and incidental movement over the course of a day. Pedometers can also help to motivate you to become more active by offering you feedback. A recent study looked at what would happen to overweight, inactive women if they accumulated 10,000 steps every day for 8 weeks. The results were lowered blood pressure and improved glucose tolerance, which reduces the need for insulin and helps prevent fat storage. What's more, using a pedometer to measure their total steps increased their daily activity levels by 85%.

Living it

Clip a pedometer onto your trousers and measure how many steps you take each day. Aim for at least 10,000 steps each day to lose weight, although you should build up to this figure over a month or two if you are very unfit or very overweight. It's also beneficial if you can include a non-stop walk each day of 4000–6000 consecutive steps, which equates to approximately 30–40 minutes of exercise.

Day 115 tip – Motivation and mindset

Keep a food diary of everything you eat for at least three days

Whether you are just starting a new eating plan or want to get a better picture of your current diet, the process of writing down exactly what you eat and drink can be very helpful. It increases your commitment and awareness and encourages you to eat better. A food diary allows you to identify patterns in your eating habits, such as your portion size, what meals work best for you, and what time of day you are most likely to stray.

Living it

Bite it and write it. Draw up a page or design a spreadsheet with columns that highlight your breakfast, lunch, dinner and snacks. For each meal, write down what you ate, how the food was cooked and your portion size. You can also leave a space to make comments about how you felt, how hungry you were, and how many glasses of water you had. Keep a food diary for at least 3 days and include a weekend day to get the most accurate picture of your diet.

Day 116 tip – Good food

Cut 400 kilojoules (100 calories) a day from your diet

Genuine long-term weight loss is most likely to occur when you make small and progressive lifestyle changes, which then develop into permanent habits. One such change is to reduce your energy intake by just 400 kilojoules (100 calories) a day. This may not seem like much, but it will make a big difference over time. That can add up to 6 kilograms of body fat per year. Now there's one small change you can stick to and build on.

Living it

Here are seven easy ways you could cut your kilojoule intake down each day. Adopt one today, or mix and match so you do at least one on each day of the week.

- Eat one less chocolate biscuit.
- Have one less full-cream milk latte or cappuccino.
- Have one less stubby, can of beer or glass of wine.
- Have a single scoop of ice-cream instead of a double scoop.
- Have a thin sausage instead of a thick sausage.

- Eat one slice of bread less.
- Have steamed asparagus instead of mashed potatoes with your dinner.

Day 117 tip – Move more
Look after your existing muscle tissue

Muscle is the most active, kilojoule demanding tissue in your body, working continuously to burn fuel. It's like the engine of your body and the bigger your engine, the more fuel you'll burn (especially when you press the accelerator and exercise). When you fast or crash diet and cut back your kilojoule intake severely you can lose muscle tissue, which slows down your metabolic rate. You need to avoid dietary strategies that can potentially break down muscle tissue.

Living it

Cutting back your kilojoule intake is only effective if you combine it with other strategies that compensate for the slowdown in your metabolic rate. Eating plenty of lean protein and performing regular cardiovascular exercise can help to minimise the muscle loss associated with a lower kilojoule diet. Resistance training is also beneficial, helping to protect muscle tissue and actually increase muscle density.

Day 118 tip – Motivation and mindset
Replace old negative habits with powerful new behaviours

Habits are an automated response to a stimulus that you make without thinking, and you may have a few that are affecting your weight. Could you drink a little less alcohol with dinner, cut back on junk food on Friday nights, or have a few less biscuits with your coffee? Old habits can die hard, but you can distance yourself from them by creating new ones. For example, instead of watching TV, go for a walk or do things around the house in the ad breaks instead of munching on potato crisps.

Living it

Breaking old habits and forming new ones is one of the more challenging aspects of fat loss, but here is a method to improve your chances of success. Identify a limiting factor, and think about what new behaviours you can install that will ensure your old habit is dumped. Reinforce your new behaviour, allow for the odd setback and don't go back. Creating new habits requires repetition before they become automated rituals, so keep at it.

Day 119 tip – Good food

Eat a healthy dinner. It's the most likely meal to be stored

Do you normally have a big dinner? Some diet experts argue that it doesn't matter when you eat and that it's what and how much you eat that's important. While I agree it's important to focus on quality and quantity, there is some research to say that when you eat can have an impact on your body shape. A study comparing identical meals found that those who ate the meal at night lost less weight (–4.4kg) over a one-month period compared to people who ate the same meal earlier in the day (–7.3kg). Research has also shown that overweight people are more likely to consume more of their kilojoules later in the day. Following are some helpful guidelines for your evening meal.

- Make your dinner low in fat, with small portion sizes.
- Dinner is an ideal time to get your 4–5 servings of water-rich vegetables.
- Substitute part of your servings of rice, pasta and bread with water-rich vegetables.
- Minimise your alcohol intake with dinner.
- Use dinner to balance your day. When you have had fatty treats during the day, have a clear soup or light dinner. Alternatively, eat well during the day when you are going to have a fatty dinner.

Living it

Try to consume the greater proportion of your kilojoule intake earlier in the day. Any food consumed at night is more likely to be stored because your kilojoule-burning rate, or metabolism, is naturally lower.

Day 120 tip – Move more

Vary your intervals to maximise results

I've already mentioned that interval training is a great way to burn more fat and up the intensity of your training. But to maximise your results, make sure you gradually progress with the ratio of your intervals to rest periods. There's no magic timing between the interval and rest, but it's important to make adjustments as your fitness improves. Studies have shown that an 8-second interval followed by a 12-second rest period is beneficial, but the study was on unfit beginners on a stationary bike. Shorter intervals are also better suited to exercise equipment, where you have a clock in front of you.

It's not so practical to look at your watch twice every 20 seconds when you're walking or cycling outside.

Living it

As your fitness improves, gradually increase the sprint period, and reduce the rest period when you do interval training. You'll also need to adjust the ratio of work to rest, depending on the activity. For example, walkers would need a shorter rest period than runners because walking is a much lower intensity activity. Swimmers might also find laps more practical than time. For example, swim two laps of freestyle then swim a slow recovery lap of breaststroke.

Day 121 tip – Motivation and mindset

Learn how underweight people gain weight, then do the opposite

While there are many people who struggle to lose weight, there are others who find it just as hard to gain weight. Being underweight can be just as detrimental to your health as being overweight, and underweight individuals are advised to eat more kilojoules than their body uses for fuel. Dietary advice to gain weight includes:

- Have large snacks between meals
- Drink lots of kilojoules
- Eat energy rich foods
- Eat at the slightest hint of hunger
- Eat more than normal by increasing your portion sizes
- Eat before bedtime
- Use large quantities of dietary supplements.

Living it

Take a good look at these tips and learn what *not* to do if you want to lose body fat. Following these strategies makes you gain weight or may have caused weight gain in the past, so make sure you take the opposite path.

Day 122 tip – Good food

Five simple dinner swaps to make those kilos drop

The kilojoules you eat at night are most likely to be stored. But you don't want to go to bed hungry.

Living it

Continuing on in this series of tips, here are five small things you can do at dinner to cut back your kilojoule intake without having to go hungry.

Instead of…	Go for…	Save…	Comments
Rice (1 cup) = 920kJ	Steamed veggies (1 cup) = 220kJ	700kJ	Extra veggies instead of rice cuts your kilojoule intake significantly; you can also do this in Asian restaurants
Cheddar cheese (60 grams) = 1110kJ	Fetta cheese (60 grams) = 760kJ	350kJ	When making a salad or your own pizza, fetta tastes great and has less fat
Potato bake (average serve) = 1100kJ	Baked potato = 460kJ	640kJ	Ditching that cream and cheese seems easier when you're saving over 600 kilojoules; keep the skin on your baked potato for extra fibre
Chocolate cake (average serve) = 1450kJ	Fruit salad and low-fat ice-cream (average serve) = 600kJ	850kJ	If you like dessert after dinner, this swap makes a massive difference
Pasta and cream sauce (average serve) = 3500kJ	Pasta and tomato sauce (average serve) = 1600kJ	1900kJ	Halve your pasta portion and add extra vegetables for an even bigger saving

Day 123 tip – Move more

If you're too tired to exercise, do some exercise

Do you often feel too tired to exercise? There are many reasons why you may feel fatigued, including poor diet, lack of sleep and a variety of medical conditions. But it can also be laziness, inactivity and a lack of fitness that makes you tired. If you rule out a medical condition for your fatigue, feeling too tired to exercise might be the best possible indicator that you need to exercise to have more energy. Aerobic exercise makes your heart stronger and more efficient, elevates mood and improves the quality of your sleep. Ultimately, these all result in more energy and less fatigue. Saying you're too tired to exercise is really one of the worst excuses you can use.

Living it

Very few things can perk you up and boost your metabolic rate like exercise. Try exercising in the morning if you feel too tired to exercise at the end of the day. Make sure you include activities you enjoy to maximise your motivation to want to exercise, no matter how tired you are.

Day 124 tip – Motivation and mindset

Learn to be more optimistic

Research has demonstrated that positive people are more likely to be successful. They get better grades, win more contests and make more money. Most importantly, they also lose more weight. The main difference between optimists and pessimists is how they deal with setbacks. Optimists think a setback is temporary, limited in its effect and not entirely their fault. Pessimists do the opposite, seeing the setback as permanent, far-reaching and all their fault. Understanding the difference between optimism and pessimism is important because both tend to be self-fulfilling prophecies. For example, pessimists see setbacks as permanent, so they tend to give up more easily.

Optimistic people see a setback as temporary, so they're more likely to do something about it, and because they take action the setback becomes temporary.

Living it

Is your glass half-full or half-empty? There are varying degrees of optimism and negativity, and most people fall between the two extremes. But you can learn to be more optimistic. When you suffer a setback in your lifestyle changes, assume it's temporary and don't indulge in self-blame. Take credit when things go well, which will reinforce your new behaviour, and make the result more likely to be permanent. Optimism is a tool; a way of thinking about the good and bad things that happen to you that increases your chances of success. Why not use it when you can

Day 125 tip – Good food

Keep your glycemic load in check

The glycemic index (GI) of foods has become quite well known, but the glycemic load (GL) is relatively new and just as important. GL is a fine tuning of the GI that takes into consideration the portion size of carbohydrates and how this affects blood sugar levels. For example, consuming large quantities of a low GI carbohydrate food (such as white pasta) has a high

GL. Blood sugar levels will still rise dramatically, resulting in a spike in the release insulin to help deal with it. Alternatively, eat a small portion of a high GI food, and your GL will remain low, and you're blood sugar won't spiral out of control. Technically, you can calculate the GL by taking the GI of a food and multiplying it by the quantity of sugar in a serving (GI x grams of carbohydrate per serving). It is a measure that incorporates both the quantity and quality of the dietary carbohydrates consumed.

Living it

Don't worry too much about the science or let this confuse you. Basically, the glycemic load stresses the fact that you need to eat both suitable 'types' and 'amounts' of carbohydrates to effectively control blood sugar and reduce the need for insulin. Portion size still counts, even if the food is low GI. The glycemic load is just another tool to help you eat better and direct you towards a style of eating that is most likely to help you lose weight.

Day 126 tip – Move more

Make time for exercise, no matter how busy you are

A lot of overweight people are too busy to exercise. Lack of time is said to be the number one barrier that stops people from increasing their activity levels. Yet most adults watch at least 3–4 hours of TV each week. While I agree that there's never enough time to do everything, there is always enough time to do the most important things. The choice then becomes yours as to what are the most important things. Is anything more important than your health?

Living it

It's not so much a lack of time but a lack of priority. Doing other things instead of exercise is a choice. If you struggle to find the time to be active, the following strategies can help you prioritise exercise and weight loss.

- **Make an exercise appointment with yourself** – Plan your exercise sessions in advance and record them in your diary. Identify a time that best fits into your day without disrupting other activities.

- **Use your time well** – Work out as hard as you can and burn off the maximum amount of kilojoules that you can in the time you invest in exercise.

- **Hire a trainer** – A personal trainer will help keep you committed. When you have money invested and someone waiting for you, it's more likely you'll exercise.

Day 127 tip – Motivation and mindset

Don't be in denial. Make sure you are doing enough to get results

If you want to lose weight and fat, the results you achieve will ultimately depend on what you actually do and not what you might think you do. Are you really exercising five to seven times per week, and is your fat and alcohol intake consistently under control? You see, the more overweight you are the more likely you are to underestimate how much you eat, and overestimate your physical activity. You'll also underestimate your weight by a few kilos. A study of one group of dieters showed they ate 4200 kilojoules more than they recorded in their food diaries and burned 1000 fewer kilojoules than their exercise records indicated. Four out of five people from all age groups and body shapes believe they eat less and exercise more than they actually do. This behaviour is not conscious and has also been identified to a lesser extent in lean subjects. But this would have more impact on people who are overweight, especially those who are frustrated at their lack of results.

Living it

Be aware that it's very common to underestimate how much you eat and overestimate how active you are. Use a watch to measure your physical activity, and once in a while check your daily fat intake.

Day 128 tip – Good food

Make your bad choices better

Healthy eating means making good food choices most of the time and unhealthy choices less often. Another way to improve your diet is to make better choices when you need to indulge. This can reduce the damage on your healthy eating plan.

Living it

If you must treat yourself, try to minimise the damage.

Instead of ...	Go for ...
Large French fries	Small French fries
Two glasses of wine	One glass of wine
Block of chocolate	Individually wrapped chocolate

Instead of ...	Go for ...
Large glass of fruit juice	A small glass of juice and a glass of water
Regular cola	Small cola
Fatty dessert	Share your dessert, and halve your portion
Garlic bread	Fresh roll with a little butter or olive oil
A large slice of cake	A sliver of cake

Day 129 tip – Move more

Incorporate exercise into your work life

If you have an inactive job, you can try to compensate for all those idle hours by incorporating exercise into your work life. The workplace environment has a very strong influence on the ideas, attitudes and lifestyle of most working adults, and is a great setting to promote better health. Healthier staff are a great asset to any business, with reduced absenteeism and improved productivity.

Living it

Does your workplace support a healthy lifestyle? Following are some ways you could incorporate more physical activity in your workplace.

- **Ask your boss** – See if your boss would be interested in improving the health of all staff. Some examples of successful corporate health programs include health and fitness assessments, subsidised or free memberships for fitness clubs or gyms, provision of health and fitness equipment, showering facilities or volleyball courts at the work site, lunchtime sporting events, walking clubs, regular seminars or health newsletters for employees.

- **Do it yourself** – Look for ways you can be active before or after work, or in your lunch break. You can also look for ways to accumulate movement throughout the day, like walking to get a sandwich at lunch or volunteering to go to the bank. You could even show some initiative and form your own walking group with your work colleagues.

Day 130 tip – Motivation and mindset

Realise that you can say no

Do you find it hard to say no? Do you make personal sacrifices because you don't like to let someone down? It may seem hard when you hear things like 'I made this cake especially for you', or 'forget your walk, let's go for a coffee'. But to really get results, you might have to place yourself first occasionally. Don't say yes to everyone and everything, otherwise it becomes impossible to give yourself fully to anything, including the things that matter most. If you dish out your energy in smaller and smaller servings, you'll get back smaller and smaller rewards.

Living it

Reflect on what's important, and take control. Time is not abundant. Prioritise the things that matter and start saying no to the rest. Don't automatically say 'yes' when someone places demands on your time. Learn to say 'no' and put the focus back on the things that are important to you, like healthy eating and regular exercise.

Day 131 tip – Good food

Modify your recipes to help you lose weight

Although there are many excellent low-fat cookbooks available, it is often very easy to adapt your own favourite recipes to fit into your low-fat lifestyle.

Living it

It's easy to substitute high-fat, high-kilojoule ingredients with healthier choices that don't sacrifice taste or texture. The table below offers some helpful ideas.

Instead of ...	Go for ...
Coconut milk/ cream	Canned evaporated skim milk and/or plain low-fat yoghurt mixed with 1–2 tbsp desiccated coconut; mix ½ coconut milk with ½ evaporated skim milk
Cream	Evaporated skim milk, plain low-fat yoghurt for sauces; blend 250g ricotta cheese with 1 tbsp sugar for cream with sweet dishes
Cream cheese	Ricotta cheese blended with a little castor sugar and vanilla essence; light cream cheese

Instead of ...	Go for ...
Hard cheese	Reduce quantity, use fat reduced block cheese; use ½ low-fat grated cheese and ½ breadcrumbs/rolled oats for toppings
Shortcrust pastry	Filo pastry, use half quantity of pastry, line bottom or top only
Sour cream	Cottage cheese or ricotta cheese blended with a little lemon juice; add mustards, garlic and herbs for a tasty topping for vegetables

Day 132 tip – Move more

Lift weights in addition to cardiovascular exercise, but not instead of it

Performing a combination of resistance training and cardiovascular exercise is an effective way to train for weight and fat loss. But it's important to consider your primary training goal and find a balance between the amount of cardio and resistance training you do. You'll be much more likely to get results if you focus on one specific goal. Resistance training shouldn't take the place of cardiovascular training, especially if you have a lot of fat to lose. If your waist measurement is over 101cm for men, and over 91cm for women, cardiovascular exercise is the best investment of your time. Don't even contemplate weights unless you are doing cardiovascular training at least 5 days a week. If you don't have as much to lose, you can afford to devote more time and energy to resistance training. A final consideration is variety and motivation. If you get bored just doing cardio and you find weights keeps you focused and interested in exercise, you could also argue for its inclusion in your training program.

Living it

Keep your strength training intense but short in duration (20–30 minutes). Limit it to two or three times a week and still try to do cardio on those days. That way you can maximise the time and energy you put into your cardiovascular fat-burning exercise.

Day 133 tip – Motivation and mindset

Be your own cheerleader

There will be times when the only support team you have is yourself. Try not to depend on others to make you feel good about your achievements. The reaction of other people is something beyond your control. You are in the best position to deal with yourself when things aren't going so well.

Living it

Be kind to yourself and treat yourself like you would a friend. Celebrate your progress and try not to obsess about setbacks. If you are struggling for motivation, sit down and collect your thoughts. Remind yourself why this is important to you, and the consequences of inaction. Don't forget to remind yourself of what you have already achieved, and even the benefits that may be a little harder to measure like better sleep, better health and just feeling better about yourself.

Day 134 tip – Good food

Give fizzy drinks the flick

One of the worst choices you could make to quench your thirst is soft drink. Loaded with sugar, kilojoules and bone softening phosphoric acid (it makes the fizzy bubbles), you get absolutely no fullness or nutrients with all those nasties. One typical can of soft drink contains 10 teaspoons of sugar, which would take between 20 and 30 minutes of walking to burn off. Energy drinks and flavoured mineral waters can be put in the same category. Research has shown a clear link between soft drinks and obesity. People who consume more soft drink take in more kilojoules, eat less fruit and are more likely to be overweight.

Living it

Don't buy it, don't drink it, don't have it when you're out. Drink water and skim milk instead. If you must drink soft drink, aim to have less than you are having now. The diet varieties are obviously much lower in kilojoules, and are a better choice if you want to lose weight and body fat. However, I worry about the long-term consequences of artificial sweeteners and encourage you to only have them in moderation.

Day 135 tip – Move more

Exercise with your family

Don't use your children as an excuse not to exercise when you can involve them in your new lifestyle. With the rate of childhood obesity skyrocketing, it's important to set a good example, and get your children involved in physical activity. Spend quality time together doing something active, not just sitting around a table eating.

Living it

Choose from the following activities, depending on the age of your children:

- Get a carry-pouch and take your baby out for a long walk; you can both enjoy the scenery and the extra weight will give you a better workout
- Take your baby or toddler for a brisk walk or run in their stroller
- Walk to the local park, playground or school with your child
- Go to a park and kick a ball, fly a kite or throw a frisbee with your older child
- Plan an active family weekend outing such as canoeing or bushwalking with your teenage child.

Day 136 tip – Motivation and mindset

Focus on your health and wellness, and weight loss will come

Yes, I know that weight and fat loss is probably your focus, but it's hard to continually stay motivated for something negative. In fact, the drive to lose body fat in overweight people can be surprisingly low. While there may be a strong desire to lose weight, the commitment to change habits and take action is often small. This may be because of low self-esteem after a number of failed weight-loss attempts. It's also possible there are aspects to your work life, social life, private life and family life that have contributed to you having more body fat than you'd like. The sooner you prioritise some changes to your lifestyle and attitude, the sooner you'll get results. Try to orientate your thinking and focus on improving your health and feeling better, not just losing weight. Improving your health will add value back to all other aspects of your life, including your energy, longevity, virility and productivity. And when you have those things, weight loss will be a lot easier to achieve.

Living it

To succeed at fat loss, lifestyle changes have to become a major priority in your life. Don't wait until illness or disease makes it an urgent priority.

Day 137 tip – Good food

Don't eat more of a food because it's low fat

Don't be fooled by the labels. Just because something is 97% fat free doesn't make it a weight-loss miracle food. A number of products like yoghurts, cakes, ice-cream and biscuits are labelled 'low fat', yet they still can have significant amounts of sugar and kilojoules. Other foods such as reduced-fat cheese, light milk and light sour cream are still very high in fat. Research has shown that there is also a tendency for people to consume larger portions of fat reduced foods, or consume additional full-fat foods afterwards. People who received a yoghurt labelled 'low fat' consumed more energy during their next meal than people with a nutritionally identical yoghurt labelled 'high fat'. This suggests that information about fat content was more influential than their normal fullness response.

Living it

While it's important to cut down on dietary fat, some low fat, fat free and reduced-fat foods are still high in kilojoules. Low fat eating is only one piece of the puzzle. Don't eat larger portions of a food just because it's a healthier choice. Foods with a high moisture content can also be confusing because they may have a low fat content by weight (due to the water) but still be extremely high in fat.

Day 138 tip – Move more

Get hold of some puppy power

Dogs can be extremely motivating and supportive workout partners for walkers and joggers. Their enthusiasm is contagious, they're ready to go in an instant, and they're persistent about wanting to get out for some activity. Research has shown that dog owners are generally more physically active and report higher levels of physical fitness than non-dog owners. If you don't want to own a dog, I'm sure a neighbour or friend would be happy to offload Rover for an hour or two.

Living it

Including dog walking as part of your exercise routine will bring health benefits to both of you. Just don't rely on dog walking as your only source of exercise for weight control, as you'll need to include activities that are more intense. Make sure you both get plenty of water after your adventures.

Day 139 tip – Motivation and mindset

Use affirmations that inspire you

Affirmations are short, authoritative statements that you can repeat to yourself when you're mood is down, and to adjust any limiting beliefs. They are similar to self-talk, except affirmations are short statements rather than a whole language. Affirmations can become a powerful motivating force through repetition because our emotions, perceptions and actions are shaped by our most dominant thoughts. What we most often tell ourselves is more likely to become self-fulfilling prophecy. Just as positive affirmations can be influential, so can negative ones. For example, repeating statements like 'I'm so unco-ordinated' or 'I can't do it' can actually lower expectations of yourself, and reinforce bad habits. Over time, these affirmations can result in a negative, overweight self-image and self-destructive behaviour. Fortunately, you have the capacity to change how you think and use more positive affirmations to help motivate you.

Living it

Encourage your thinking habits to work for you, not against you. Increase your awareness of any negative affirmations you say repeatedly to yourself and dispute them. Replace them with positive thoughts that motivate you. Try to find one or two short statements that you can call on when you need to. Look at some motivational quotes or think about any advice you've been given that has always stuck with you. One of my online coaching clients likes to use 'nothing tastes better than being thin', while I personally like 'a quitter never wins' when I'm trying to push myself during exercise. The key is to find something short and repeatable that really means something positive to you.

Day 140 tip – Good food

Take advantage of the surprising benefits of calcium for weight loss

A study where subjects ate two cups of yoghurt a day to increase their calcium intake showed that the participants lost an average of 5 kilograms over 12 months. Their findings showed that:

- calcium-rich diets help your body turn more kilojoules into heat than into body fat
- calcium-rich diets contribute to fat loss in the stomach area
- calcium-rich diets prevent muscle loss in dieters
- calcium-rich diets can help minimise midlife fat gain.

These benefits were not the same when the study participants used calcium supplements. It's thought other components in low-fat yoghurt, such as high quality protein, may also offer benefits.

Living it

Calcium can do more than just strengthen your bones. Aim for three to four servings of calcium-rich foods per day to accelerate weight loss, making sure to choose the lowest fat varieties of dairy products. You can also get calcium from non-dairy sources such as green leafy vegetables and canned fish.

Day 141 tip – Move more

Don't let age be a barrier. It's never too late to start exercising

Not only can exercise help to energise you and burn fat, physical activity can prevent and even reverse about half of the physical decline normally associated with ageing. Much of what we consider normal signs of ageing is just muscle wastage from inactivity. Due to increasing life expectancies, we now have many quality years for travel, leisure and recreation. Exercise has also been proven to help with other aspects of your health that become more important as you get older, such as upper and lower body strength, hip and shoulder flexibility, agility, balance and co-ordination.

Living it

If you rest, you rust. Muscle doesn't know age; it only knows use and disuse. The older you get, the more you can benefit from exercise to counteract the muscle loss associated with ageing (and inactivity). Staying active can also prevent weight gain as you get older. It's never too late to start.

Day 142 tip – Motivation and mindset

Don't blame your genes

You often hear people blame their excess body fat on big bones or genetics or inheritance, and there is a strong link between your body shape and the weight of your parents. But this link is just as much about environment as it is genetics. According to a study on identical twins where the siblings had different activity levels, only 6% of the most active twin was overweight, compared to 37% of the more sedentary twin. While your genes may have an influence on your metabolism, this is not a life sentence for excess body fat.

Living it

Recent increases in obesity have been occurring much too rapidly to be explained by changes in the gene pool. You can inherit 'fat' genes from your parents, but of more concern is when you inherit their bad habits, such as a poor diet and lack of exercise. These lifestyle factors have a more important part to play in weight gain. That's good news because you can do something about them. Genetics are something you can't change so don't get too caught up on it. You can still overcome 'bad' genes with good health.

Day 143 tip – Good food

Put your fridge on a diet

What's inside your fridge? A good portion of the food you eat and drink will come out of your refrigerator, so make sure it's in good shape to help you get into shape. Having healthy foods always at hand makes healthy eating easier.

Living it

Take a good hard look at what's inside your fridge and freezer and see if it needs a makeover. Check expiration dates and throw out anything that's old enough to vote. Even frozen foods have a shelf life. Substitute high-fat foods with low-fat versions, have sauces and herbs to dress up healthy foods, and pre-cut fruits and vegetables so they are available quickly and easily. Here are some healthier choices to support your healthier lifestyle.

Instead of ...	Go for ...
Full-fat yoghurt	Low-fat natural yoghurt
Full-cream milk	Skim milk
Butter or margarine	Dijon and grain mustard, horseradish
Soft drink, fruit juice	Water jug
Yellow cheese	White cheese like cottage and ricotta
Salami, bacon, Devon	Lean ham, smoked chicken breast
Sausages	Lean meats and seafood
Milk chocolate	Mixed raw nuts
Alcohol	Lots of fresh herbs and vegetables
Cream	Eggs
Ice-cream	Sorbet

Day 144 tip – Move more

Enjoy a round of golf, but don't use it as your only source of exercise

One way to add a little variety to your walking routine is to play golf. A game of 18 holes equates to about 7 kilometres of walking. While it's too 'stop-startish' to be ideal for fat burning, it's an enjoyable form of low intensity exercise. One study found that playing 18 holes of golf burns around 1900 kilojoules (450 calories) per round, and participants who played three times a week lost approximately 1.5 kilograms over 12 months without any change in diet.

Living it

While the weight-loss benefits are minor, golf can still burn off excess kilojoules and is a fun and social addition to your exercise routine. Try to walk quickly between shots and minimise stoppages to maximise fat burning. A word of warning, however; the benefits of golf will quickly evaporate if you use a powered cart or if you finish with a few high-kilojoule drinks in the clubhouse afterwards.

Day 145 tip – Motivation and mindset

Have a goal weight (conditions apply)

It's common for people to have a goal weight that is meant to be ideal for their height, or an old mark they want to get back to. Firstly, your height has nothing to do with your weight. Measuring your weight as a ratio of your height (BMI) is irrelevant on an individual basis (it's best used to help scientists compare population groups for obesity). It's also difficult to compare your weight between the past and the present or use it as a future goal because you lose muscle and bone density as you age. Ironically, the best way to prevent the loss of muscle and bone density is to perform resistance training, which can actually make you gain weight on the scales.

Living it

While it's important to have a goal, body weight is not a good target to aim for. Instead of a striving for a goal weight, have a 'goal to wait'. Wait for at least 3 months before weighing yourself. Wait before constantly jumping on the scales. Women should also aim to weigh themselves at the same time of their menstrual cycle because changing fluid levels can cause their weight to fluctuate by up to 3 kilograms a month. It's nice to see the scales coming down, and they will in time but don't get too caught up on a goal weight as an indicator of your long-term success.

Day 146 tip – Good food

Eat your greens

Your mum probably told you to eat your greens, and she was right. Not only are green leafy vegetables low in kilojoules, pound for pound they provide more calcium than milk, more iron than beef, about as much vitamin A as carrots, more vitamin C than oranges, generous quantities of the B group vitamins, zinc, magnesium and various other minor nutrients. Eating plenty of high nutrient foods like green leafy vegetables helps both your insulin levels and metabolism function at their best, which in turn helps with fat loss.

Living it

Look for ways to include more lettuce, broccoli, broccollini, cabbage, spinach, bok choy and pak choy in your diet. They only need minimal preparation and cooking time, and can even be eaten raw in salads. They are also great as a side dish, in soups and stir-fries.

Day 147 tip – Move more

Adjust your exercise plans according to your mood

There is concrete evidence to prove that exercise helps boost your mood and decrease anxiety, with some psychologists even prescribing it as a strategy to help deal with depression. But that's when you've actually finished exercising. To get yourself out of a rut, consider modifying your planned training or activity to better suit your existing mood.

Living it

Here are some recommended activities to suit different moods.

Mood	Best activity	Comments
Anger/ frustration	Strength training or boxing	Both are great outlets to disperse your aggression in a positive way.
Sad or depressed	Long walk, yoga	Choose calming activities. You could even try an indoor bike while listening to some relaxing tunes.
Bored	Swimming, tennis, bushwalking, paddling	Just as your body can reach a plateau, so too can your mind. Try exercising in a different place, or add something new to your routine.
Tired/ unmotivated	Anything for 10 minutes	There will always be days when you're tired and there seems to be a mountain of excuses piling up. The old you would have stayed in bed. Why not just go anyway, but take it really easy. Sure, it's better to go for 40 minutes, but 10 minutes is still worth it and you'll have that sense of achievement.

Day 148 tip – Motivation and mindset

Live by the 10 commandments (of fat loss)

Among all the mixed messages and conflicting information there are a few golden rules that ring true. You could call them the 10 commandments of fat loss, and they have stood the test of time. They are supported by sound scientific research and they are the tips you'll see virtually all diet experts agree on.

Living it

Try to adopt these 10 commandments and live by them every day:

1. Burn off more kilojoules than you consume
2. Drink more water
3. Move more
4. Eat more vegetables
5. Don't diet or deprive yourself
6. Keep your portion sizes down
7. Eat fewer processed foods
8. Eat low GI carbohydrates
9. Always eat breakfast
10. Restrict your alcohol intake.

Day 149 tip – Good food

Control your food cravings

A food craving is a strong desire for a specific type of food that people often go to some lengths to satisfy. The foods craved are often high in sugar, fat and kilojoules (chocolate, cake, ice-cream) and they can be a big distraction when you are trying to lose weight or reduce your kilojoule intake. Cravings are a learned behaviour in response to a stimulus, such as an emotion, hormones, blood sugar imbalance or the time of day. You also learn to crave the relaxation and pleasure you feel when you've eaten these comfort foods. Cravings are not your body's way of telling you that you need some specific nutrient.

Living it

Following are some tips to help you overcome or even unlearn common food cravings.

- Only eat the foods you crave when you are full. That way, you'll be content with less.

- Chew slowly to really taste and savour every mouthful of your foods, especially treats. By doing so, you'll need less quantity to be satisfied.

- To help stabilise your blood sugar levels and reduce cravings, eat low glycemic index foods, eat three meals and two small snacks a day, and make sure to eat plenty of protein and fibre. Don't go more than 4–5 hours without food.

- Once you have a food craving, try to wait 5 minutes before giving in to it. Distract yourself with another activity or go for a short walk. If the craving continues, have a small portion, or find a healthier alternative.

- Drink plenty of water, which can help to suppress your appetite by keeping your stomach full between meals and take the edge off hunger.

Day 150 tip – Move more

Train to get that exercise high

You've probably heard of the runner's high or exercise addiction. Some have described it as a state of euphoria, while others describe it as a myth. So does it exist, and how do you get it? There are several theories on why people feel good after exercise. One theory is that endorphins are released, producing a sense of wellbeing and blocking the brain's pain receptors. Another theory states that exercise serves as a distraction from other stresses in your life.

Living it

There is good evidence to suggest that exercise improves your mood and reduces stress. It's not exactly clear how, but what is certain is that it gives you a sense of achievement. You are bound to feel better about yourself when you are actively doing something about excess body fat, improving your health and gaining control. So the key is to just get out there and do it.

Day 151 tip – Motivation and mindset

Don't let your friends undermine you

Are your friends making you fat? It's not uncommon to find social situations where you are encouraged to celebrate with food or drink. They may not realise it but friends can sabotage your new, healthier lifestyle with some gentle persuasion or a few discouraging words. They may be jealous of your dedication to lose body fat or feel guilty if they indulge in a treat on their own. Research has shown that women who dine in the presence of others almost double the amount of food they eat compared to when they eat alone. People eating in groups of friends also tend to eat more than those in groups of strangers. This could be partially due to distracted eating or reduced willpower around friends.

Living it

When trying to lose weight be wary of friends who continually offer you fatty foods or try to pull you away from your exercise program. Explain to them how important this is to you, and that you need their encouragement. Arrange gatherings with friends that don't necessarily revolve around food, such as bushwalks or time at the beach.

Day 152 tip – Good food

Eat more vegetable and legume dips

There are not many better ways to enjoy vegetables and legumes than with a tasty dip. Dips are very versatile and very easy to prepare. Be wary of creamy dips that contain soft cheese such as French onion.

Living it

Dips can last for several days in the fridge, so they can be on hand for a quick snack, entree, finger food, a filler, a replacement for butter on a sandwich, a pizza topping, in salads, or as a light meal with bread. You can serve dips with cut vegetables such as capsicum, cucumber, celery, carrots, mushrooms, lettuce rolls or snow peas. They also work well with crusty wholemeal bread, dark rye bread, multigrain cruskits and crackers, and toasted pita bread. Here are some of the popular vegetable and legume dips you could buy or even make yourself:

- Tomato salsa (with chili, garlic and onion)
- Chili con carne dip (mashed kidney beans, chili, tomato and garlic)
- Humus (only add a small amount of oil and tahini with the chickpeas)
- Eggplant dip, or baba ganoush (only add a small amount of oil and tahini)
- Beetroot and mint (use a low-fat yoghurt)
- Roasted red capsicum with sweet chili dip (add a small amount of crushed almonds).

Day 153 tip – Move more

As your fitness improves, push yourself a little harder

If you are beginning to breathe a little easier during exercise, you can actually be going backwards. The fitter you get, the more efficient your body gets at moving you around. This is because you may weigh a little less, your leg strength improves and your lungs can extract more oxygen from the air. This also means you'll burn fewer kilojoules when you exercise. A study on participants who lost 20% of their body weight found they used 35% fewer kilojoules compared to an identical workout they did before losing the weight.

Living it

Unless you continue to progress and up the duration, intensity or frequency of your exercise, your results will grind to a halt. So don't just plod along with the same old routine. Keep a record of any training information you can (distance, duration, kilojoules used, steps taken) so you've always got a mark to improve upon, and you'll continue to get results.

Day 154 tip – Motivation and mindset

Learn from the losers, and make their habits your own

A US study looked for common habits among thousands of people who had lost over 12 kilograms and kept it off for more than 12 months.

Living it

If you'd like to lose a significant amount of weight and keep it off, try to adopt these common traits like other successful losers.

- **Desire** – This factor was rated number one. Their desire to lose weight was stronger than their desire to overeat or avoid exercise.
- **No fad diets** – Most subjects ate several meals and snacks a day, including the odd sinful treat.
- **Daily exercise** – Most made walking or jogging a part of their daily life.
- **Train harder** – Over 80% of subjects reported that they exercised more often and more vigorously than with previous weight-loss attempts.
- **Professional help** – Most participated in some formal weight-loss program. This included regular meetings with groups, a psychologist, a dietician or a personal trainer.

- **Learn a lesson** – Every subject had failed on at least five previous weight-loss attempts. They analysed their reasons for regaining and drew valuable lessons from those experiences.

Day 155 tip – Good food

Enjoy your daily bread (conditions apply)

Bread is a high-kilojoule food, yet it can provide fullness and nutrition or fat-storing excess depending on a few variables. Wholegrain varieties of bread are by far and away the best choice because they are highest in fibre. They are more filling, so you need fewer kilojoules to feel satisfied. The fibre also slows down absorption of wholegrain bread, so it's a better source of long term energy and it reduces the need for insulin, which in turn prevents fat storage. Wholemeal is the next best choice, followed by high fibre white bread. Try to minimise your intake of white bread. It has less than half the fibre content of multigrain bread, so you'll either eat more or eat more later.

Living it

Minimise butter or margarine on your bread, and choose low GI multigrain varieties or breads made with different grains such as rye and pumpernickel. Keep your portions under control because it's easy to overeat processed grain foods like white bread.

Day 156 tip – Move more

Snack on exercise instead

Just as you might look towards a small snack of food to give you an energy boost or improve your mood, why not use exercise to do the same. Short 'snacks' of activity can distract you when you're tempted to indulge and help keep hunger pangs at bay. Who knows, after you finish your exercise snack you may not feel like that food snack. But even if you do, at least you've pre-burned a few extra kilojoules. Short snacks of exercise can also help to break up periods of inactivity, such as sitting at a desk or watching TV, and to make sure you do something on those days when you're extremely busy. You can even use them to heat you up a bit during the colder months of the year.

Living it

While these exercise snacks shouldn't replace your formal exercise program, they can be a handy addition. Look to this list below for exercise snack suggestions:

- Go for a 5–10 minute power walk

- Do some vigorous housework, like cleaning a few windows
- Ride a bike to the shops
- Walk up a few flights of stairs
- Park your car some distance from your destination
- Do some gardening
- Hop on your exercise equipment.

Day 157 tip – Motivation and mindset

Don't go it alone. Consider professional help

It's a lot harder to take this journey by yourself. Fortunately, there are many services available that can make things easier. Dieticians can help you to design a healthy eating plan, while an exercise physiologist or personal trainer can help you with your exercise program. Psychologists can help you deal with the emotional issues surrounding food, while weight-loss classes and programs enlist group support. A fat loss coach takes a broader approach, working on your food, exercise and motivation to maximise your chances of getting results.

Living it

I genuinely believe that if you follow the advice in this book, you'll achieve lasting weight and fat loss. But the more support you can muster, the better. If you haven't used professional help in the past, why not try a new angle. It could be just the kick-start you need. Regular contact with a health professional who specialises in weight control can provide motivation and up-to-date information.

Day 158 tip – Good food

Gain control over insulin to accelerate weight loss

You might think that insulin is only relevant for diabetics, but its role in weight control is significant. After eating foods containing carbohydrates, your body breaks them down into glucose for absorption. When your blood sugar levels rise, the body releases the hormone insulin to help glucose pass from your bloodstream into the body's cells, where it's stored or used as fuel. If you are overweight or inactive, the cells gradually develop what's called insulin resistance, so your body needs to crank out more insulin to do its job. This might all seem okay, but too much insulin has a few negative effects on your waist and hips because it:

- converts and stores glucose into body fat

- triggers the storage of dietary fat as body fat
- prevents your body using stored body fat as fuel.

A recent study found that people who secreted high insulin levels had a far more difficult time losing weight than those who secreted low levels of insulin.

Living it

You can speed up weight loss by minimising the need for your body to release insulin and by increasing your body's sensitivity to insulin. You can do this by:

- eating more low GI foods and fewer high GI foods
- being active, which helps to reduce blood glucose levels
- keeping your portion sizes under control, which lowers the glycemic load
- minimising foods high in both sugar and fat, such as cakes, biscuits, pastries, ice-cream and chocolate
- eating more foods with less processing to maximise their fibre and nutrient content.

Day 159 tip – Move more

More reasons to move more in the morning

I've already described how exercising before breakfast burns more fat (see day 93) but there are additional weight-loss benefits to consider.

- It boosts your metabolic rate at the start of the day, before you've eaten.
- It helps to regulate your appetite for the day.
- You're more likely to be consistent with your exercise because you'll be less likely to put your exercise off for other interruptions.
- It's a real 'pick me up' and makes you feel energised for the rest of the day.
- It sets a good precedent and creates a healthy mindset, which can boost your desire to eat more healthily for the rest of the day.

Living it

While making the time to do your cardiovascular exercise is the most important factor, there are some advantages to working out in the morning. Even if it's only on the weekends, try to find the time to do a few morning workouts each week.

Day 160 tip – Motivation and mindset

Make your home a health farm

Make sure the environment where you spend most of your time supports your new lifestyle. It can make a world of difference to live in a home where you don't have to face temptation every day. You can't rely on willpower all the time.

Living it

Following are some tips on how to make your home a healthier environment.

- Avoid bringing junk foods or unhealthy treats into your home. **You can't eat what you don't have. Save your indulgences for when you eat out occasionally.**
- Have a bowl of fresh fruit prominently displayed in your kitchen.
- Use notes and inspirational photos on your fridge to help keep you motivated.
- Purchase or hire some exercise equipment for regular use.
- Stock your pantry and fridge with lots of tasty, healthy foods.

Day 161 tip – Good food

Eat more low energy density foods

The energy density of a food (also called kilojoule density) is the number of kilojoules per gram. High energy density foods give you lots of kilojoules per mouthful, while low energy density foods such (fruits and vegetables) have the least amount of kilojoules per serving. One study declared that energy density is the key food issue influencing weight, especially the lack of fullness obtained from high-kilojoule density foods.

Living it

Try to focus your diet on low energy density foods like fibrous vegetables, such as spinach, broccoli, capsicums and zucchini. It's a great way to feel full while still reducing your kilojoule intake. Also, watch your portion sizes of nutritious, energy dense foods, such as nuts, avocados and extra virgin olive oil.

Low energy density	Medium energy density	High energy density
Vegetables, fruits, brown rice, grilled chicken, kidney beans, wholemeal pasta with tomato-based sauce, steamed fish, natural low-fat yoghurt, porridge	White bread, low-fat vanilla ice-cream, tuna salad sandwich	Butter or margarine, oil, chocolate, pizza, peanuts, cheese, cheesecake, potato chips

Day 162 tip – Move more

Lift weights before your cardio workout

Do you perform your cardiovascular exercise before or after you lift weights? It does make a difference, and there is a strong case for doing your resistance training first. A recent study showed that of the two groups who performed an identical cardio and weights workout in a different order, the weights then cardio group used 10% more fat as fuel. The kilojoule use was virtually identical but the proportion of fat used as fuel was higher. This is because the body tends to use glucose as fuel early in a workout and also during intense, short-burst exercise such as resistance training. By doing weights first you'll deplete your stored glucose levels, increasing the likelihood of burning body fat during your cardiovascular exercise.

Living it

Perform resistance training before your cardiovascular exercise to maximise fat burning. Just make sure you still perform a cardiovascular warm-up for 5–10 minutes before lifting weights to prevent injury.

Day 163 tip – Motivation and mindset

Learn from the past

I'm sure you have made more than one attempt to lose weight in the past. So what can you learn from those experiences so you don't repeat the same behaviours that didn't work last time? Losing weight permanently will usually involve leaving behind old and destructive habits, and replacing them with new and healthier ones. This won't be easy, but unless you change it's just another case of 'if you always do what you always did, you'll always get what you always got'.

Living it

It's not really a mistake until it happens again. We all make mistakes, but it's the learning from them that's important. When did you last really enjoy exercise, and why? What healthy recipies do you remember enjoying. Did weighing yourself motivate or de-motivate you? Try to learn from your weight-loss, exercise and diet history, and modify your behaviour for the future.

Day 164 tip – Good food

Eat differently to the opposite sex

Have you ever wondered why your partner or friend of the opposite sex loses weight at a different rate to you? If you eat most of your meals with your partner of the opposite sex, it's advisable to do a few things differently. Women especially need to adjust to a slower metabolic rate, a higher percentage of body fat, a stronger hunger response after exercise, and a closer link with emotional eating.

Living it

The following table highlights some of the differences between men and women in regards to diet and weight control.

For men	Dietary focus	For women
5–6 meals a day	Meal frequency	4–5 meals a day
Moderate	Portion size	Small
A little more	Alcohol intake	A little less
High	Protein needs	Moderate
Low risk	Emotional eating	High risk
Moderate demands	Healthy fats	High demands
Moderate	Hunger after exercise	Strong

Day 165 tip – Move more

Use your local park as an outdoor gym

Most people have a local park within fairly close proximity of their home, which provides an excellent venue for a wide range of outdoor exercises. Some parks even have a fitness course, with several exercise stations along the way to target your major muscle groups and add variety. Whether your nearby park is small or a full-sized playing field, why not take advantage of the fresh air and open spaces and burn some kilojoules in the process.

Living it

Try some of these activities in your local park:

- Walking and running on the grass

- Sprint and interval training
- Find a bench and do step-ups, dips and elevated push-ups (feet on bench, hands on the ground)
- Do body weight circuits on the grass, combining cardio with push-ups and lunges
- Take along some friends and throw a frisbee. You could also play a sport like volleyball, soccer, softball, cricket or touch football
- If it's a big park, time yourself doing 3–5 laps so you can try to beat it next time.

Day 166 tip – Motivation and mindset

Monitor and improve your self-talk

Language has a powerful influence on your behaviour. Self-talk is your own personal language, including the internal dialogue you have with yourself that reflects your beliefs, attitude and thoughts. These thoughts can influence your mood, energy and behaviour by making you feel confident or nervous, motivated or discouraged, depending on what you say to yourself. Improving the way you communicate with yourself can make a difference.

Living it

Many people are careful about how they communicate with others but give little thought to how they communicate with themselves. Negativity breeds stress and failure, but once you recognise negative self-talk, replace it with objective and encouraging thoughts. When you find yourself using negative self-talk, take a deep breath, say 'stop' to yourself and think about other possibilities, solutions, or explanations. Give recognition to your strengths and be kind to yourself when things go wrong. As you become more aware of your self-talk, experiment by saying more positive things to yourself. Play a few mind games and see what works. Below are some practical examples.

Instead of ...	Go for ...
I look huge in this.	I'm making changes and heading in the right direction.
I'm too fat to exercise.	
I'm too busy to exercise today.	I'll exercise at my own pace.
I can't keep exercising this hard.	I need to squeeze in a short walk today.
It's too unpleasant outside to exercise.	Just a few more minutes.
	How can I exercise indoors today?
I don't like too many vegetables.	Where can I find some tasty vegetable dishes?
I'll never be as good as them.	I'm working on beating my own personal best.

Day 167 tip – Good food

Learn to minimise hunger

Hunger and appetite have a strong influence over your body shape. The hungrier you are, the more you'll eat; however, learning to control hunger and appetite is very important when you are trying to reduce your kilojoule intake. Hunger is the natural drive to find and eat food and it's characterised by stomach discomfort, tiredness, increased intensity over time, and it cannot be relieved by distractions. Appetite is more psychological and it can be in the absence of hunger. It can be brought on by the expectation of food, by smell or the time of day.

Living it

There are several factors that increase and decrease hunger and appetite.

Things that increase hunger	Things that decrease hunger
Caffeine and alcohol	Water
Cold temperatures	Warm temperatures
Dietary fat	Fibre
Inactivity	Exercise
Salt	Protein
Low blood sugar	Eating slowly

Day 168 tip – Move more

Exercise as hard as you can for as long as you can

An interesting study looked at how much fat was used during 30 minutes of exercise at two different levels of intensity. One group of subjects trained at 50% of their aerobic capacity (a measure of fitness), while a second group exercised at a higher level of exertion, or 70% of their aerobic capacity. You can see the results in the table below. The low intensity exercise group used a higher proportion of fat as fuel (50% vs. 40%). But the higher intensity group burned more fat (9.1g vs. 8.1g) because of the greater amount of total kilojoules used (865), even though the proportion of fat use is lower. The higher intensity exercise will also help to boost metabolic rate to a greater extent both during and after exercise, improving cardiovascular fitness and burning more kilojoules.

	50% aerobic capacity	70% aerobic capacity
Total kilojoules used	613	865
Intensity	light–moderate	high
Fat utilisation as fuel	50%	40%
Kilojoules of fat used	307	344
Grams fat used	8.1	9.1

Living it

These results suggests that if fat loss is your goal then exercise at the highest intensity you can tolerate, for as long as you can continue to exercise. That way you'll maximise fat and kilojoule burning and boost your metabolic rate to a greater extent.

Day 169 tip – Motivation and mindset

Get enough sleep. It really can help you lose weight

Do you often wake up tired and wish you had had more sleep? Sleep quality and quantity has an important role to play in determining your success at weight and fat loss. A study on 24 identical twins found that the fattest twin was more likely to have sleep problems and snored more than their leaner sibling. Poor sleep will result in tiredness and fatigue, which can alter your eating patterns and reduce your energy levels. This can make it harder for you to stay motivated and stick with your lifestyle changes. It can also slow down your metabolic rate, keeping your kilojoule-burning rate sluggish even if you are eating well and exercising. Sleeping less also means extra waking hours for eating, which could further increase your kilojoule intake.

Living it

To improve your sleep habits, try to apply the following tips.

- Keep to a regular sleep schedule
- Avoid caffeine and alcohol before bed
- Sleep in a cool, dark, quiet room
- Plan your day the night before (to reduce thinking and worrying in bed)
- Avoid depending on sleeping pills
- Use relaxation techniques
- Be active.

Day 170 tip – Good food

Eat more whole grains

Whole grains are known to help in the fight against fat, but there is a little uncertainty about what they actually are. Whole grains, in their natural state, contain all the original parts of the entire grain seed, just as they would grow in a field. Foods made from the whole grain that have been processed (cracked, crushed, rolled, lightly pearled or cooked) can only still be considered whole grain if they contain the same rich balance of nutrients found in the original wholegrain seed. Examples of some well-known grains include barley, brown rice, buckwheat, bulgur, corn, oats and rye. Some lesser known whole grains include quinoa, sorghum, spelt and wild rice. Processed grain foods that have the bran and/or the germ removed (white bread, white pasta, white rice) have significantly less nutritional value. With most of the fibre and nutrients gone, the concentrated kilojoule component of the grain elevates the GI, making these foods less than ideal for fat loss.

Living it

Less processing makes these foods higher in nutrients and more filling and therefore good for fat loss. If you are a little unsure how to find or prepare whole grains, consider the following tips on how to include more whole grains in your healthy eating plan.

- Enjoy wholegrain salads like tabouli.
- Choose wholegrain varieties of breads and rolls.
- Include brown pasta and rice in your evening meals.
- Search the Internet for wholegrain recipes and ideas.
- Have high fibre breakfast cereals made with whole grains, such as whole wheat, oats or barley.

Day 171 tip – Move more

Re-test your fitness

Let's check how your cardiovascular fitness is going. While this book is focused on helping you to lose fat and keep it off, the fitter you become the better your body is at burning fat as fuel. And we all want that.

Living it

Remember way back on day 24 when I encouraged you to walk for 3–5 kilometres and write down how long it took you to complete? Well today is the day for a re-test. Go out and do the exact same course, the identical distance that you completed many moons ago. Depending on how you're reading this book, make sure there is at least 3 months difference between your two test dates. Hopefully this time you are fit enough to finish it sooner. You can record your details from day 24 here, and also note your new information.

	Benchmark (day 24)	Re-test
Date		
Course distance/ description		
Time to completion		
Heart rate 60 seconds after completion (optional)		

What do my results mean?

If you bettered your time, well done. Your body has a higher capacity to process oxygen and is therefore a better fat burner. You are fitter, hopefully leaner, and feeling better for it. If you stayed the same or fell back a little, it's not the end of the world. Spend some time reviewing some of the exercise strategies throughout the book, and see where you could make improvements.

Day 172 tip – Motivation and mindset

Stop making excuses, and find a way

There's always an excuse why people can't exercise, can't push themselves hard today, can't change their diet yet, can't drink less alcohol this weekend, can't find the time, can't get out of bed early this week, and don't feel motivated. For some people trying to lose body fat, making excuses is often their greatest barrier to success. Excuses are fattening. But for every excuse there is an alternative or solution, another way to make the sort of choices that will improve your health and make a difference. If there are 10 reasons why you can't do something and one reason why you can, focus on why you can.

Living it

If you don't want to do something, you'll find an excuse, but if you really want to do something, you'll find a way. If you want results, find a way to get out of the excuse making mindset. Put your energy into finding solutions rather than making excuses.

Day 173 tip – Good food

Eat slower to accelerate your weight loss

This might seem so simple, but it is amazingly effective. It's well known that it takes 15 to 20 minutes for your stomach to signal that it's full, so if you eat slower, you'll eat less in that time. Just look at this great little study. Two groups were asked to eat a tomato-based pasta until they were comfortably full, although one group was asked to eat quickly and the other to eat slowly. The fast eaters ate 2713 kilojoules in 9 minutes, while the slow eaters consumed 2432 kilojoules in 29 minutes. The fast eaters consumed 10% more kilojoules in a third of the time. Imagine how this could stack up over three meals. The fast eaters also reported feeling less satisfied and hungrier an hour later. Just don't confuse slow eating with distracted eating, where you eat too much over a long period of time because you are focused on other things.

Living it

Eating rate affects your kilojoule intake and your fullness level, so slow down and savour the flavours and textures of your food. Some useful strategies to help slow down your eating include:

- Use a small spoon or utensil
- Take small bites
- Chew your food thoroughly
- Put your utensil down between bites
- Drink water between mouthfuls
- Serve a small portion so you have to get up for more
- Serve drinks in small glasses.

Day 174 tip – Move more

Watch less television, or exercise in front of it

How much TV do you watch? Time spent watching TV is directly associated with obesity, and as television viewing hours increase so do the chances of being overweight. One study found that people who watch more than three hours of TV a day were twice as likely to be obese than those who watched less than an hour a day. Another study showed that

66% of adults could not find the time to exercise, yet they all watched three or more hours of TV a week (some over three hours a day). Television has a number of effects that actually cause an increase in fatness. It decreases the amount of physical activity that you could be doing, slowing your metabolic rate and increasing your body's capacity to store fat. It can also slow down your metabolic rate. A study on children showed that the metabolic rate of those watching television was lower than those who were reading. Television viewing seemed to place the children into a trance-like state, slowing down their body's natural rate of kilojoule use.

Living it

The simple fact is this: the time you spend watching TV could be time spent exercising. The average Australian watches around 22 hours of TV a week, so by substituting some of that time for exercise, you can make a massive difference to your body shape. Try to limit your TV viewing time unless you have completed your physical activity for the day. If you would find it hard to watch less TV, find a way to exercise in front of it.

Day 175 tip – Motivation and mindset

If your results plateau out, make additional changes

A plateau is a period of stabilisation in weight and fat loss when your body begins to adapt to your new lifestyle. Your results will come to a halt as your body adjusts to your new levels of exercise, healthy eating and metabolic changes. This happens because your body gradually makes it harder to lose body fat by lowering your metabolism as you lose weight, increasing your appetite as you eat fewer kilojoules, and reducing the kilojoules used during exercise. A plateau can occur at any time as you lose body fat, and can last for weeks or months. It's important to note that plateaus should be expected because it's not possible to lose fat continually.

Living it

To get off a plateau, you need to make additional changes above and beyond those that triggered your early results.

- **Reduce your kilojoule intake** – A body that weighs less requires less fuel, so gradually cut back your kilojoule intake. You can reduce fat, sugar and alcohol more, spread your kilojoule intake out more over the day, try spicier foods, eat less at night, eat a wider variety of foods, and have smaller portions.

- **Increase your kilojoule expenditure** – Vary your type of exercise and increase the intensity, duration and or frequency. Do more spontaneous movement at your home or work.

Day 176 tip – Good food

Identify if you are an emotional eater

For some people, learning about healthy eating and cooking will be enough to help them improve their diet, while for others there are additional emotional issues that will need to be addressed. Emotional eaters use food to regulate mood, cope with stress or overcome feelings of anxiety or boredom. Because the type of foods used to deal with negative emotions are usually unhealthy (alcohol, chocolate, chips, ice-cream, cake), emotional eaters often find it hard to lose body fat. Over time, a very strong bond can form between certain foods and certain emotions.

Living it

Feelings of sadness, anger, stress, guilt or frustration are a part of life, and how you deal with these emotions can have a big impact on your body shape. Answer yes to any of the following questions, and you may be an emotional eater. Becoming aware of your emotional eating is the first step in addressing it.

- Do you eat when you're bored?
- Do you eat when you're not hungry?
- Do you have feelings of guilt or self-loathing after overeating?
- Do you continue to eat after you are full?
- Do you eat alone out of embarrassment at your large portions?
- Do you eat alone out of embarrassment at the type of food consumed?

Day 177 tip – Move more

Find time for some Fartlek training

Another way to add variety to your exercise routine is to incorporate Fartlek training. It might sound a little on the nose, but Fartlek is actually Swedish for 'speed play' and it's similar to interval training except that your sprint intervals are unstructured. Because there is no predetermined schedule to follow, you can work to your own interval lengths and pace, and respond to how you're feeling on the day. Just like interval training, Fartlek helps you boost your kilojoule burning and aerobic fitness, and lose weight at a faster rate than steady state training. It's also a great way to prevent training boredom and get over a weight-loss plateau.

Living it

Instead of using time as a measure of your intervals, Fartlek training is random. If you are out walking, running or cycling, you can incorporate short, high intensity bursts between parked cars, trees or lampposts as a marker. You could even sprint along the straight sections of road, and walk round the corners or up the hills to recover. You can also use it paddling or swimming, by alternating between slow, medium and fast speeds. Get creative and make up your own adventure. Because there is no set pattern, your training time passes a lot quicker because every workout is different.

Day 178 tip – Motivation and mindset

Use motivational quotes and affirmations to help inspire you

Have you ever seen images of an athlete's fridge or bathroom mirror, plastered with post-it notes full of motivational messages and uplifting sayings? Why not use them yourself. In a society that condones overindulgence yet condemns the effects, we are constantly bombarded with messages to eat this, or sit down and do that. Quotes are a great way to get motivated and help you to stay focused on your goals.

Living it

'If it is to be, it's up to me'. Why not surround yourself with messages that inspire you and drive you towards a healthier, leaner future. Find quotes that mean something to you and relate to your circumstances. If you'd like to see some of my favourite motivational quotes, I include one with each weekly edition of my free weekly email newsletter the Better Body Update. Just go to <www.andrewcate.com> and click on the free newsletter link to subscribe.

Day 179 tip – Good food

Eat a wide variety of foods

Having the same foods over and over again can actually reduce your exposure to vitamins and minerals, and slow down your rate of fat loss. Food variety is a relatively new concept in nutrition, increasing your awareness of how many different types of foods you eat. Eating a wide variety of foods exposes your body to a wide variety of vitamins, minerals and nutrients, helping your metabolism function at its best. There is even some research to suggest that new foods take more kilojoules to break down and digest because your body isn't used to them. And you don't need big portions to benefit.

Living it

Try to eat at least 30 different types of food each day, and 40 different types of food each week. Plant foods are the best source of vitamins and minerals, but no single food supplies all the nutrients you need. A balance of the five food groups will give you the best variety and help to maximise your metabolism.

Food group	Examples
Grain foods	Breads, cereals, crispbread, rice, crackers, oats, muffins, crumpets, bagels, pasta, couscous and potatoes
Fruit and vegetables	All fruits and vegetables – fresh, frozen and canned
Milk and dairy foods	Try to have low-fat varieties: milk, yoghurt, fromage frais, cheese – hard, soft, cottage cheese
Meat, fish and alternatives	Beef, pork, lamb, eggs, poultry, fish, beans and pulses, nuts and seeds
Fats and oils	Small portions of predominantly plant-based fats, such as olive oil, avocado, nuts and seeds

Day 180 tip – Move more

Cool down after exercising, especially if your training was intense

The better you feel after exercise, the more likely you'll be to want to do more. So if you want to prevent soreness after your activity, a cool down is important, especially if you have done a hard workout or performed interval training. Studies have shown that a cool down is more effective than stretching at preventing post-exercise muscle soreness. Continuing to move at a slower pace helps your body to adjust from an active state to a resting state, preventing soreness and cramps. Muscle contractions actually help to squeeze blood back to your heart, which prevents blood pooling in your lower body. This also helps to prevent varicose veins.

Living it

Continue your activity at a lower intensity for 5–10 minutes, or until your heart rate is less than 100 beats per minute. Avoid coming to a sudden stop after your activity, which can cause dizziness or faintness. If your activity is light in intensity and short in duration, you only need to cool down for a minute or two. However, if your training is intense, focus on a good cool down and stretch the predominant muscles used in your activity.

Day 181 tip – Motivation and mindset

Use your weekends to get ahead, not behind

Do you have a pretty healthy routine during the week only to blow it by eating and drinking to excess on the weekends? Just 2 or 3 days of overindulgence and under-exercising can really set you back. Recent studies have shown that most people tend to take in more kilojoules on Fridays, Saturdays and Sundays. As the weekend approaches, people tend to exercise less and reduce their fruit intake while at the same time increasing their intake of takeaway food and alcohol.

Living it

You can still enjoy yourself, but try to minimise the damage. Take advantage of the extra time you have away from work by getting outside for a longer workout or doing some vigorous gardening. You can also use the time to get organised with your food by planning your meals for the week, and pre-making some batches of food for freezing.

Day 182 tip – Good food

Don't skip meals. It can actually make you fat

Skipping meals was a strategy commonly used in the seventies to help people lose weight. It didn't work then, and it won't work now. It can actually make things worse. Firstly, it can slow down your metabolic rate. When you limit your kilojoule intake too drastically, the body alters its metabolism, reducing the amount of kilojoules you burn. It will also make you hungry, so you'll crave high-kilojoule foods, lose your willpower, and increase the likelihood of bingeing later.

Living it

Skipping meals is not a good way to reduce your kilojoule intake. To keep your metabolism firing and reduce hunger, men should eat something about every 3 hours and women every 4 hours. Be especially careful not to skip breakfast, which boosts your metabolism and encourages your body to burn fat.

Day 183 tip – Move more

Don't hibernate over the winter months

Do you have a plan to combat the natural tendency to store fat over winter? It's easy to put off exercise until tomorrow when it's cold and dark outside. But sticking to a regular fitness routine is vital if you wish to lose weight or stay in shape. While the colder weather may test your motivation, exercising through winter offers its own unique benefits. Exercise in colder temperatures actually increases the amount of fat used as fuel, so you'll be in better shape when spring and summer come around. It also improves your mood, sleep and energy levels, keeping those 'winter blues' at bay. Below are some suggestions on how to stay active through winter.

- **Join a gym** – You'll find a wide range of equipment in a comfortable environment.

- **Indoor activities** – Sports such as basketball, volleyball, badminton, squash, cricket, soccer and netball may all have indoor competitions in your area.

- **Purchase/hire exercise equipment** – Exercise while watching TV in the comfort of your own home.

- **Exercise videos/DVDs** – There is a wide range of videos and DVDs. Look for cardio-based shows that elevate your heart rate.

- **Get out there** – There's no reason you can't exercise outside. Just make sure you dress in layers, wear a hat to prevent heat loss in extreme cold, and keep your fluids up.

Living it

Don't lay idle just because it's cold. There are plenty of choices for both indoor and outdoor activities.

Day 184 tip – Motivation and mindset

Don't get confused by health information. It all depends on your perspective

With a steady traffic jam of diets, scientific studies and celebrity fads, it can be hard to know what direction to take when it comes to nutrition, fitness and fat loss. It's easy to get confused or frustrated when one week, for example, you can eat potatoes and the next week you can't. But a big cause of the confusion is the simplification of dietary advice. Generalised information in the popular media goes out to a mass audience, but this same information can be helpful for one person and misleading for the next.

For example, if someone says 'swimming is a great exercise', well that's true if you want to get aerobically fit but not so true if you want to lose body fat (see day 348 for more on swimming). The food strategies and exercise guidelines used to achieve one goal (e.g. weight loss) can be totally different to those used to achieve a different goal, such as cardiovascular fitness or muscle strength and tone.

Living it

There is no 'one-ideal-program-for-all', and any health advice needs to be tailored to you and your goals. This book is all about how to achieve fat and weight loss. It will show you the best foods and exercises specifically for fat and weight loss.

Day 185 tip – Good food

Cut back on or cut out butter and margarine

Have you ever wondered what is the best option between butter or margarine for weight loss? The best choice is a spread with the least amount of kilojoules. That being the case, the best spread is to have neither. Butter and margarine are virtually pure fat, containing a massive 11 grams of fat per tablespoon. Both are extremely high in kilojoules and should really be minimised if your goal is to reduce body fat. They are also high in the type of fat that is a poor choice for your heart. If you only have a small amount of butter or margarine occasionally, make your choice based on taste, and enjoy in moderation.

Living it

Look for alternative spreads like low-fat cream cheese, spreadable cottage cheese, low-fat mayo, chutney, relish and pickles. If you can't bear the thought of life without fatty spreads, check the nutrition information panels and choose one with a lower fat and kilojoule content.

Day 186 tip – Move more

Don't overeat because you've exercised

Do you feel ravenous after a workout? The effect of exercise on your appetite varies according to the activity type, the intensity and your gender. Exercise can temporarily lower your appetite right after your activity, but some people get hungry. Your level of hunger after exercise is important because you don't want to undo all your hard work with an uncontrollable urge to eat. Women tend to experience greater levels of hunger after exercise, as their bodies try harder to maintain existing fat stores for survival of our species (childbirth and lactation). Appetite is also partially regulated by temperature control. If you feel hot after a hard workout, you may experience a greater drop in appetite. However, if you are cool, such as after swimming, you may feel ravenous.

Living it

More intense exercise is thought to have the greatest appetite suppressing effect, so include intervals in your workout to really warm you up. Make sure you also drink plenty of water after exercise because dehydration can make your body crave food. Exercise can influence hunger differently in people, so experiment to find out what's best for you.

Day 187 tip – Motivation and mindset

Live like you've already lost it

Have you thought about the lifestyle that you'll need to live if you are to achieve lasting fat and weight loss?

Can you see yourself living the kind of life that you want to live? See yourself with the type of health you want, a pantry with the right type of foods and a room full of exercise equipment. Why not start living that way now.

Living it

Start to think and live like someone who has already got the results you seek. Regular exercise and healthy eating are the habits of lean people. Why not make them your own? Here are some healthy habits you can adopt today:

- Seek out new healthy food ideas and recipes
- View exercise as a pleasure not a burden
- Solve problems without turning to food
- Encourage others to be healthy
- Always have a water bottle with you
- Have a pantry and fridge stocked with healthy foods.

Day 188 tip – Good food

Use avocado instead of butter or margarine, but don't go overboard

Avocados are extremely high in fat, but are they a good choice for weight control? Yes and no. Avocados are high mono-unsaturated fats, which is the type of fat that is least likely to be stored, and also good for your heart. A recent study revealed that a group of people on a kilojoule-controlled diet who used avocado instead of other fats (butter/margarine, cheese, cream cheese, full-fat dairy) lost body fat. The study proves that avocados are a healthy substitute for other fat sources, and are less fattening. However, the subjects were on a kilojoule-controlled diet. Because avocados have an extremely high-kilojoule content, enjoy them in moderation.

Living it

When you have a salad sandwich, use a scraping of avocado instead of butter or margarine. A small serve of avocado on toast or cracker bread with cottage cheese, grilled tomato and cracked pepper also makes for a good breakfast or snack. Just keep you portion size small.

Day 189 tip – Move more

Wear the right shoes for your activity

One essential piece of exercise equipment is what you wear on your feet. Footwear that is correctly fitted and designed specifically for your activity can make your exercise more enjoyable, and prevent injury. On the other hand, inappropriate, ill-fitting or worn-out shoes can cause blisters, corns, calluses and foot problems such as heel and arch pain, stress fractures and Achilles tendonitis.

Living it

When you are shopping for exercise shoes, keep the following tips in mind.

- **Ignore the brand and colour** – Good fit, support and cushioning are more important than appearance, popularity or celebrity endorsements.

- **Buy activity specific shoes** – No single pair of shoes is right for all activities. Running shoes focus on cushioning, ball sports have more focus on lateral stability, while walking shoes need more flexibility from the heel to the toes.

- **Know your feet** – Everybody's feet are different, and some brands suit some people more than others. Get to know any special requirements your feet have, such as your injury history and arch height.

- **Replace worn shoes** – Shoe wear depends on your foot anatomy, body weight, type of exercise, frequency of training and the training surface. If you use them regularly, most shoes will lose their cushioning within six to 12 months, which can place the jarring back on your knees and ankles.

- **Others** – Some other important considerations are to wear the socks you'd wear during your activity, try on both shoes, try different brands so you can compare, and make sure they feel comfortable from the start. Exercise shoes shouldn't need to be stretched or broken in.

Day 190 tip – Motivation and mindset

Forget these fast fix fraudsters

We've all seen the infomercials. In just 5 minutes a day, the latest gadget or sit-up device will rid the world of fat, with just four easy payments. And don't forget the steak knives. Unfortunately, all is not what it seems, as you would probably expect, and maybe learnt when you purchased something like this before. There is no simple solution to weight loss and just because a product is for sale doesn't mean it's effective, or safe for that matter.

Living it

Here are five gadgets that fail to live up to the weight-loss promises they make. Save your money, but have a good laugh at their expense.

- **Magnetic ear clips** – Research on ear clips and acupressure wrist devices have shown they are totally ineffective. They hurt your ear but don't reduce hunger or cause weight loss.

- **Tummy trimming sit-up devices** – Abdominal exercises don't help you lose weight around your tummy. You need cardiovascular exercise to burn body fat.

- **The weight-loss patch** – Delivering drugs by the skin might seem revolutionary, but it's just another gimmick. The patches are available over the counter, so the drugs they administer can only have a minimal effect otherwise they would need to be prescribed.

- **Sauna suits** – Wearing a suit that makes you sweat will help you lose weight on the scales, and may even live up to the claims of 2 kilograms in 24 hours, but none of it will be fat. The loss of weight is from a loss of fluids, leaving you tired, dehydrated, and susceptible for fast weight regain next time you have a drink.

Day 191 tip – Good food

Only snack if you reduce the size of your main meals

Do you consciously eat less lunch and dinner on the days you snack? Snacking can actually increase your total kilojoule intake (and your weight) if you don't reduce the portion size of your main meals. The weight reducing benefits come from eating smaller, more frequent meals – which is known as grazing. It helps to spread your kilojoule intake over the day, so your body is more likely to use up fuel as you go rather than storing it. In addition, digestion itself burns kilojoules, so by eating more often you'll burn more kilojoules. Some useful snacking guidelines are:

- Have a second breakfast as morning tea
- Try to eat a little less at lunch and dinner
- Avoid snacking before going to bed at night
- Drink plenty of water to prevent hunger between meals
- Eat low GI and human interference (HI) foods to maximise fullness and help you to feel satisfied with smaller portions.

Living it

Instead of eating three large meals each day, aim for five mini meals to really kick-start your metabolic rate. Try for a small snack between breakfast and lunch, and again between lunch and dinner.

Day 192 tip – Move more

Breathe deeper during exercise, and in everyday life

Stored body fat needs oxygen to help it burn (be used as fuel). More oxygen means more fire, and more fire means more fuel is burnt. For this reason, the way that you breathe is important for weight control. Shallow breathing doesn't allow your body to process oxygen efficiently. Research has shown that many people use less than 25% of their lungs' capacity. On the other hand, deep breathing can increase the amount of kilojoules you use by up to 40%. Merely increasing your oxygen intake through conscious, deeper breathing can increase your body's ability to burn fat.

Living it

Deeper breathing can boost your metabolic rate, increase your energy levels and reduce fatigue. You can do this while sitting in traffic, at your desk or standing in a queue. Try to consciously breathe deeper to maximise your oxygen intake throughout the day, and make sure you can hear your breath during exercise. Breathing is also important during weight training because you need to supply a good deal of oxygen to your muscles and brain. It's generally best to exhale during the harder, lifting, pushing or pulling phase and breathe in during the easier, lowering phase of each movement.

Day 193 tip – Motivation and mindset

Watch out for the winter blues

Bad weather and a lack of sunlight can trigger a mild form of depression known as seasonal affective disorder (SAD). One characteristic of the disorder includes a significant weight gain in the winter months, so it can have a dramatic impact on your body shape. Other characteristics of SAD include a lack of energy, increased frequency and quantity of food, longer sleep and fatigue.

Living it

People who live in countries with more extreme changes in seasons are more likely to suffer from this condition, but it still can have a mild impact on Australians. To reduce the chances of SAD causing you to overeat and to feel fatigued over the winter months, try to consciously spend some time outdoors in the fresh air, especially if there's a succession of grey days.

Day 194 tip – Good food

Five simple snack swaps to make those kilos drop

A simple swap that cuts out just 400 kilojoules a day can add up to around 3.5 kilograms less body fat a year.

Living it

Here are five small things you can do between meals to help reduce your kilojoule intake.

Instead of ...	Go for ...	Save ...	Comments
Guacamole (3 tbsp) = 1080 kilojoules	Salsa (3 tbsp) = 60 kilojoules	1020 kilojoules	Guacamole has good fats but a lot of kilojoules; salsa is a great alternative
Peanuts (50 grams) = 1285 kilojoules	Pumpkin seeds (50 grams) = 930 kilojoules	355 kilojoules	Snack on seeds for a lower-kilojoule nutrient boost

Instead of ...	Go for ...	Save ...	Comments
Room temperature water = 0 kilojoules	Cold water = 0 kilojoules	40 kilojoules	Your body uses up to 40 more kilojoules to reduce iced water to body temperature for absorption
Potato crisps (50 grams) = 1050 calories	Apple = 200 kilojoules	850 kilojoules	While fruit is high in natural sugars, any fruit is a better choice than crisps
Café latte (1 cup) = 325 kilojoules	Skinny cappuccino (1 cup) = 120 kilojoules	205 kilojoules	Watch the sugar and treats you have with your coffee

Day 195 tip – Move more

Don't worry about muscle turning into fat if you stop lifting weights

Have you heard that if you gain a little muscle from strength training and then stop, the muscle will turn into fat? This is a classic health and fitness myth. Can skin turn into bone? Of course not, and neither can muscle turn into fat. Muscle and fat are two completely different tissues, and it is physiologically impossible for one to convert into the other. However, the ratio between fat and muscle is very important for both physical fitness and body shape. Resistance training will increase the density and strength of your muscles. It will boost your metabolic rate and increase your appetite. If you stop lifting weights, the muscle shrinks, just like a limb that's been immobilised in a plaster cast. If you don't lower your kilojoule intake (stopping weights will slow down your metabolic rate, and reduce your kilojoule needs), the excess fuel will be stored as fat. While it may appear that muscle has turned into fat, the muscle gets smaller and the extra kilojoules are deposited as fat in the areas once occupied by muscle.

Living it

Inactivity can cause muscle cells to shrink and fat cells to expand. To prevent this from happening, stay active, or if you can't do that, eat less.

Day 196 tip – Motivation and mindset

Treat any underlying medical condition that may be causing your excess body fat

Although rarely the primary cause, there are a number of medical conditions that may contribute to a person being overweight. These can include hypothyroidism, polycystic ovarian syndrome, depression, chronic tiredness (sleep apnoea), chronic pain, chronic gastrointestinal discomfort, Cushing's syndrome, or binge eating disorder. There are also some medications, such as steroids and anti-depressants, that increase your appetite and may lead to a weight gain.

Living it

You cannot treat obesity until you treat the cause. Excess body fat can be related to other health problems, which need to be treated before weight loss can occur. Discuss any concerns you have with a doctor, who can test to see if there are any underlying medical conditions affecting your weight.

Day 197 tip – Good food

Eat more oats

One of the tastiest, cheapest and healthiest ways to eat more whole grains is to have more oats. From a fat loss perspective, the soluble fibre in oats attracts fluid and fills you up, giving you long-lasting energy, and minimising the need for the sugar and fat storage hormone insulin. Studies have shown that oats maintain normal blood sugar levels longer than most other foods. Oats are also a good source of fibre, protein, vitamins, minerals and healthy fats.

Living it

Eaten as muesli in summer, porridge in winter, or even added to soups and smoothies, oats are versatile and delicious. Avoid the commercial crunchy (toasted) mueslis that are baked in fat and the pre-flavoured varieties that are high in sugar. Make your porridge with skim milk and water, and sweeten with berries, sultanas, banana, peaches, low-fat yoghurt or a little sugar or honey. You can also make your own natural muesli by adding different nuts and seeds, and a small amount of shredded coconut or dried fruits.

Day 198 tip – Move more

If you have a cold or flu, don't lie about and do nothing (conditions apply)

If you only have a head cold, with symptoms above your shoulders (runny nose, sneezing, sore throat) and you have no fever, it's okay to exercise. However, if your illness is more like a flu than a cold, including symptoms such as fever, tiredness and muscle aches then it's probably best to rest until your fever subsides. You can't sweat out a cold or flu. Exercise won't speed up your recovery. In fact, it can actually make things worse. Physical activity forces your body to focus all its energies and blood flow on your working muscles and away from your struggling immune system.

Living it

If you don't feel at your best, ease up a little on your exercise intensity, and shorten the duration of your workout. Some activities will also be better suited than others. For example, cardiovascular exercise will place extra stress on your upper airways and respiratory system, while weight training or stretching would be less taxing. You could always go for a light walk and save your energy for a more intense workout once you feel better.

Day 199 tip – Motivation and mindset

Don't use a lack of money as an excuse

People who say they can't afford to go to the gym or can't afford a personal trainer could be very surprised if they examined their budgets. It's often a lack of priority and not a lack of money that's the main barrier.

Living it

Look at these 10 strategies you could use to actually help you lose weight. Eliminate two or three that aren't relevant to you and you should still have enough money to afford a casual gym visit or a shared 30-minute personal training session each week.

Weight-loss strategy	Weekly money saved
Cut back your portion sizes at lunch and dinner	$2
Drink tap water instead of fruit juice or soft drink	$4
Walk to shops to get your Sunday paper, or at least part of the way	$2

Weight-loss strategy	Weekly money saved
Make your own healthy sandwiches on 2 days when you may have bought lunch	$5
Don't have a biscuit or cake when ordering a coffee	$3
Go for an evening stroll instead of hiring a DVD	$5
Cut your own grass, walk your own dog, wash your own windows	$5
Make your own popcorn with no butter instead of buying potato crisps	$3
Cut back on two glasses of alcohol each week	$5
Stop using butter or margarine on your bread	$1
Total	**$35**

Day 200 tip – Good food

Use your freezer to save time and kilojoules

With time in short supply these days, it makes sense to minimise your food preparation and cooking time. By using your freezer, quick food can still be good food. Knowing you have a healthy, tasty meal available for a quick reheat at home can reduce your reliance on takeaway junk.

Living it

Make sure you always have a healthy fallback meal in the freezer. Foods such as lean meats, tomato-based sauces, soups, legumes and cooked rice all freeze well. Make double batches of casseroles, pastas and mixed vegetables for the week ahead. Freeze foods in the portions you use, such as fruit, which can be added to an ice cold smoothie. If you have leftover fresh herbs, chop them finely and freeze them with water in an ice tray. You can then add them to soups and sauces. It's also good to have a supply of frozen vegetables on hand.

Day 201 tip – Move more

Try some circuit training

If you're short on time but want to build strength and burn fat at the same time, circuit training can be a worthwhile addition to your exercise routine. Many gyms and weight-loss centres offer 30 minute circuit classes, where you train on a series of weight machines for a set time (30–60 seconds) aimed at hitting all the major muscle groups. In between strength exercises, you'll often perform cardio activities like star jumps, jogging on the spot, or a short stint on a bike or treadmill to keep your heart rate up. The weights are traditionally light, so you can perform the exercises a little faster and further elevate your heart rate to maximise fat burning.

Living it

Circuit training isn't the perfect strength building or fat-burning exercise, but it's a pretty good way to achieve both things at once. Try to gradually increase the weight you lift as you progress, minimise your rest between exercises, and perform intervals where you can during the cardio component of the circuit. Try out a class at a centre near you, or make up your own circuit at home. Best results will come from doing circuit training at least twice a week in addition to more traditional cardiovascular exercise 4–5 times a week.

Day 202 tip – Motivation and mindset
Take steps to prevent middle-aged spread

There are a number of natural changes with ageing that may lead to an increase in stored body fat. Most people gain on average 5 kilograms between 35 and 45, and 1 or 2 more between 45 and 55. The most significant change is the loss of muscle mass associated with ageing, which lowers your metabolic rate. In other words, you don't need as many kilojoules to survive as you once did in your twenties or early thirties. In addition to muscle loss and a metabolism slowdown, weight gain in middle age can also be caused by:

- increased or continued eating that fails to adjust to reduced energy needs
- decreases in aerobic capacity and muscle strength
- a decrease in spontaneous physical activity or incidental movement
- lowered effectiveness of hormones that stimulate fat cell breakdown.

Living it

To some extent, the reduction in muscle mass and slowing of your metabolic rate can be overcome by regular participation in moderate exercise and resistance training. Slightly lowering your food intake to match your reduced need for kilojoules will also help to prevent middle-aged spread.

Day 203 tip – Good food

Get more vegetables, however you can

Vegetables (and fruit) can come canned, frozen and fresh, and they all are a good choice. A study has confirmed that the nutritional value of Australian canned food products is comparable to that of fresh foods. Frozen vegetables also compare well and retain virtually all of their vitamins and minerals. Depending on how long your fresh vegetables have been out of the ground, and left waiting in your fridge, frozen vegetables that are snap frozen and harvested when perfectly ripe may actually contain more nutrients.

Living it

Fresh is always best because of a slightly higher nutrient value, and lower levels of preservatives such as salt and sugar. But from a weight-loss perspective, canned and frozen foods offer convenience because they are pre-cut, peeled and easy to prepare. Use them in combination with fresh foods for best results. It may also help to get to know your local greengrocer, who may have better quality produce and a wider range of choices compared to supermarkets.

Day 204 tip – Move more

Exercise vigorously to maximise EPOC

One of the important ways that exercise helps you to lose weight and fat is by boosting your metabolic rate. However, it's not just about speeding up your metabolic rate during exercise. Another variable is for how long your metabolic rate stays elevated afterwards. This metabolic 'after burn' is called excess post-exercise oxygen consumption (EPOC), and it's the amount of extra oxygen your body needs for recovery after exercise. If you compare training to driving a car, exercise is like putting your foot down on the accelerator, where you burn lots of extra fuel. But once you take your foot off the accelerator (stop exercising), the car will still keep rolling along. EPOC is the fuel that keeps burning once you stop exercising, and it can burn an extra 50% more kilojoules than what you used up during exercise.

Living it

This is a way to continue burning more fat and kilojoules, even though your exercise is finished. Cardiovascular exercise, and to a lesser extent weight training, can elevate your metabolic rate after exercise, sometimes for up to 24 hours. How long your metabolic rate stays elevated depends on how hard and how long your workout is. The greater the intensity and the longer the duration of a training session, the higher this extra consumption of oxygen (EPOC) will be, and the longer your metabolic rate stays elevated. Of the two variables, EPOC is higher when the training's intensity increases compared to when the duration increases. In other words, long duration, low intensity training is not as effective is high intensity, shorter training sessions. Good hydration also improves EPOC.

Day 205 tip – Motivation and mindset

Use your computer to help you lose weight

If you have access to a computer, there are a number of different ways you can use it to help you lose weight and body fat. In fact, research has shown that people who use their PCs in conjunction with weight-loss programs lose three times more weight than people who don't.

Living it

Use these six suggestions to get the most out of your computer, and your weight-loss program.

1. Use a spreadsheet to monitor your diet, record you activity and track your progress.

2. Learn more about food, fitness and fat loss with the myriad diet and health related sites loaded with articles, recipes, tips, quizzes, case studies and programs.

3. Enter a chat room or check out a weight-loss blog for valuable suggestions, and join a community focused on supporting each other to achieve the same goals.

4. Subscribe to email newsletters that keep you updated and motivated each week, fortnight or month.

5. Download ebooks, fitness videos and audio programs, and purchase them online.

6. Use the services of an online trainer or weight-loss coach, who interacts with you via email. The information is tailored to your needs, and you can stay motivated at a fraction of the cost of a traditional personal trainer.

Day 206 tip – Good food

Get husky, and use this secret (dare I say miracle) weight-loss ingredient

Psyllium seed husks have been added to some breakfast cereals and meal replacement shakes. Many fibre supplements and weight-loss shakes have psyllium as their main ingredient. Psyllium is one of the richest sources of indigestible soluble fibre, which expands by up to 10 times its original volume to form a gel-like mass. You can see for yourself by putting a tablespoon of psyllium husks in half a cup of water for 20 minutes. It can help you lose weight by:

- slowing down the emptying of your stomach, helping you to feel fuller for longer
- reducing the amount of insulin needed to process blood sugar after a meal
- binding with fat and cholesterol, which is eliminated instead of being absorbed.

Living it

You can eat products that contain psyllium husks, or add them to your own foods or drinks. Just make sure you have them with plenty of water or skim milk to make you feel full. Psyllium works best in smoothies and breakfast cereals, especially when added just before serving.

Day 207 tip – Move more

Don't rely on yoga or Pilates for weight loss

Activities such as Pilates and yoga have seen a rapid rise in popularity as people seek out activities that deliver inner harmony, balance and functionality. Mind–body exercises also have wider appeal to all ages and physical capabilities. The slow and controlled movements are generally safe and low impact, yet can be vigorous enough to elicit a strength-improving response. While yoga and Pilates help with muscle strength and flexibility, it's not cardiovascular exercise and will not result in significant weight loss.

Living it

Yoga and Pilates don't make you puff enough to be effective fat-burning exercises. They are certainly better than doing nothing, but don't rely on them as your only form of activity. In combination with cardiovascular exercise and a healthy eating plan, yoga and Pilates can be part of a successful weight-loss program.

Day 208 tip – Motivation and mindset

Ditch the doona and the electric blanket

We already know that being a little bit cool speeds up your metabolism more than being a little bit hot. Considering you spend about a third of your life in bed, your temperature while sleeping is important for your body shape. When you lie in bed, it takes around two hours to heat up to the temperature you'll stay at for the rest of the night. Because you'll generally fall asleep in that time, many people will spend most of their sleep time too hot, especially if you use a doona or electric blanket. Doonas are between 3–5 times warmer than a blanket, which is why you might wake up with your feet sticking out the side of the bed as your body attempts to cool itself down.

Your body actually needs to lose heat in order to sleep well, which is mainly done through the head and face. But if your bed or bedroom room is too hot, the body may not be able to sufficiently cool itself and sleep quality can be affected.

Living it

Try to use blankets instead of a doona so you can peel off layers as you warm up. It's also best to avoid using an electric blanket, or at least turn it off before falling asleep.

Day 209 tip – Good food

Eat more soup (but avoid the creamy ones)

One of the best ways to reduce the kilojoule content of your diet and lose weight is to eat lots of soup. Ideal for lunch, dinner or even as a snack, a thick, hearty soup can be very satisfying. Soup is low in kilojoules because of its high water content, yet it's usually served hot, so people tend to eat it slowly and feel full afterwards. In fact, whole diet books have been devoted to soup. Studies have shown that a starter of tomato soup was highly successful at cutting down on subsequent food intake. Soup is also a great time saver because you can make large batches, and reheat it quickly, or freeze the leftovers. Just make sure to avoid cream-based soups that are loaded with fat and kilojoules.

Living it

Load your soup up with four of my favourite weight reducing ingredients: water, legumes, water-rich vegetables and lean meats. Add a little stock and lots of flavour with herbs, spices and condiments, and enjoy. If you have bread with your soup, avoid butter or margarine, choose wholegrain bread and keep your portions small.

Day 210 tip – Move more

Drink tea or coffee before exercise (but watch what you have with it)

Caffeine has been shown to have a role in fat loss by stimulating the hormones involved in removing fat from your fat cells during exercise. Caffeine may also boost your body's metabolic rate by 7–22%. One study found an increased metabolic rate of up to 16% 150 minutes after consuming caffeine. Another study showed runners and cyclists could run/cycle for a greater-than-normal-distance after a couple of cups of black coffee.

Living it

Consuming one or two cups of black coffee or tea before exercise will impair carbohydrate (glucose) use as a fuel, and trigger fat burning earlier. Just avoid the cream, full-fat milk, sugar, cakes and biscuits that often come hand in hand.

Day 211 tip – Motivation and mindset

Manage the hormonal changes that lead to weight gain

After the age of 45, nature starts to work against us when it comes to body fat. Women start to produce less oestrogen, while men suffer a loss of testosterone, both of which can have a huge impact on your body shape and the distribution of body fat. Women begin to transform from a pear shape to an apple shape, and also take on the higher levels of health risk that men have due to abdominal fat. Men lose testosterone at a much slower rate than oestrogen loss in women, but they can expect to gradually lose muscle mass and gain weight from a slower metabolism.

Living it

While you can't reverse all the hormonal changes with ageing and menopause, you can be pro-active and positive in your lifestyle and mindset. Gaining weight does not have to be inevitable as you age. If you do nothing, you'll lose muscle, strength and lose energy, and you'll lose bone density. But you can adopt scientifically proven strategies that will compensate for the changes taking place in your body. With a little enthusiasm and consistency you can get stronger, fitter, faster and more flexible. There's no reason why you can't maintain a healthy level of body fat at any age, and radiate with health and energy for the rest of your life.

Day 212 tip – Good food

Eat your fruit, don't drink it

Have you been kidding yourself that fruit juice is good for you? Fruit juice is promoted as a healthy and refreshing drink, and is even mentioned as a substitute for whole fruit. But this is simply not the case if you are trying to lose body fat. A glass of juice can have up to three times the kilojoule content of an equivalent piece of whole fruit, and you still won't feel as full. One glass of fruit juice has a similar kilojoule content to a glass of regular soft drink (plus a few extra vitamins). The easily digested sugars from fruit juice will be used as fuel first, making it less likely you'll burn off any other foods you have eaten, let alone the fat already stored on your body. The best choice is to eat fruit whole, as nature intended, and also drink plenty of water. Whole fruit is more filling, will give you longer lasting energy, and is more likely to help you reduce your overall kilojoule intake.

Living it

Try to eliminate, cut back on or water down fruit juice to reduce the kilojoule content of your diet. It just provides empty kilojoules without filling you up.

Day 213 tip – Move more

Understand the secret benefit of exercise

Exercise is the ultimate cure for excess body fat, and it's not just about burning off kilojoules. A consistent program of exercise will gradually increase the hormones and fat-burning enzymes in your muscles that allow your body to use fat as fuel. Exercise improves the chemistry in your body and makes your muscles demand more fat as a source of energy, even while you sleep. On the other hand, inactivity makes your muscles shrink, decreases their need for fuel and gives your body no reason to keep any fat off once you go off a diet.

Living it

Altering your body chemistry takes 8–12 weeks of consistent (at least 4 days a week) cardiovascular exercise lasting at least 15–20 minutes and leaving you lightly puffing. Be patient, but make it a priority and you will be more likely to lose weight and body fat.

Day 214 tip – Motivation and mindset

Have a laugh!

Having a good laugh is no laughing matter when it comes to improving your health. It can even help with weight loss. Not only does a good laugh help to relax the muscles in your face, shoulders, neck and upper torso, it reduces your blood pressure and stress levels. Some additional health benefits associated with laughter include:

- It is a distraction from worries to lighten stress, anxiety, depression and pain

- It requires internal exercise, where the lungs inhale and exhale rapidly, improving circulation and oxygen delivery to your vital organs

- Hormones called endorphins are released, which act as natural pain killers and help to evoke a good mood

- Catecholamines are released; they have anti-inflammatory properties and improve immune function, which may help people with arthritis or other inflammatory diseases.

Living it

Try to spend a little time with people who make you laugh. You could also watch a TV show or movie that amuses you. Laughing helps to keep your stress levels down, which can make your weight-loss journey much easier.

Day 215 tip – Good food

Improve or expand your cooking skills

The more control you have over your diet, the healthier it will be. While it will always help to make smarter choices when you are eating away from home, you can never be exactly sure how much fat, oil and sugar is in the foods put in front of you. By developing your own skills in the kitchen, you can learn how to make healthy foods taste great, prepare meals in advance and get adventurous with all those wonderful, fat-burning vegetables and legumes. You will also rely less on fast food and takeaway.

Living it

Get a hold of some healthy recipe books, or even better sign up for a cooking class. Strive to find a batch of tasty, healthy meals and snacks that you can whip up quickly and easily.

Day 216 tip – Move more

Do resistance training at home

If you're keen to enjoy the benefits of weight training but don't want to join a gym, you can work out at home. Plenty of exercises require minimal equipment or expense. Work out in front of the TV, or have some music playing to add interest and fun. Aim for two weight training workouts a week, and have 1 or 2 days' rest in between.

Living it

Following are some ideas.

- **Body weight** – Lift yourself for an equipment-free, cost-free home gym solution. You can do push-ups, lunges, dips, squats, calf raises and sit-ups with nothing more than a towel.

- **Fit balls** – You can pick these up for between $20 and $40, and they are very versatile. Search the Internet or buy a book that outlines the wide range of exercises you can perform.

- **Rubber resistance** – Rubber tubes, sheaths and sticks with straps attached can be used as a form of resistance, and to great effect. They are light, easy to use, easy to pack away, and you can even take them with you on holidays.

- **Dumbbells** – Dumbbells allow for a large variety of exercises, and don't take up too much space. You can get pre-molded dumbbells or an adjustable set that can be increased as you get stronger.

- **Exercise DVDs/books** – There are a number of books, videos, DVDs and downloadable programs on the Internet that can guide you through a basic strength training routine. It can be helpful to have a demonstration of what you are trying to do, especially if you are just a beginner.

Day 217 tip – Motivation and mindset

Recover quickly from setbacks

How do you feel when your health and fitness program falls off the rails? Do you throw in the towel and really let yourself go, or do you get back on track as soon as possible? There will be days or occasions when you overeat, drink too much, or miss the chance to exercise. A recent study looked at the difference between people who achieve their goals and those who don't. Everyone will face frustration, boredom and discomfort. There are identifiable times when setbacks are more likely to occur, such as weddings, divorce, death of a loved one, prolonged stress, menopause, festive occasions, giving up sport, quitting smoking, changing jobs and after losing weight. But what differed for those who achieved their goals was that they kept taking action when the going got tough. The non-achievers made excuses, resulting in less action and eventual abandonment of the goal. This is not to downplay the significance of these setbacks but to recognise that it's how you deal with difficult times that is crucial in determining your long-term success.

Living it

You can't change what's happened in the past, but you can change what happens in the future. Don't deliberate or focus on regrets. Don't use it as an excuse to quit. Learn from it, and get back to it as soon as you can.

Day 218 tip – Good food

Use healthy cooking methods

Cooking methods can have a dramatic influence on the amount of fat and kilojoules that end up in the foods you eat.

Look for recipes that incorporate ingredients and cooking techniques that compliment your desire to lose weight instead of working against it.

Living it

Avoid frying your food, or baking it with loads of fat. Try to use more of the cooking methods described below, which are best at capturing the flavour and nutrients of food without adding excessive amounts of fat.

- **Roast** –You can bake most varieties of meats and vegetables with minimal fat. Add pepper, garlic, herbs and spices for extra flavour. You can also cover the food to keep it from drying out.

- **Microwave** – Not only is the microwave perfect for cooking vegetables, soups and stews, it can defrost and reheat frozen foods. There are few better ways to save time and nutrients in the kitchen.

- **Stir-fry** – Stir-frying is a quick and easy way to cook vegetables and lean meats with minimal fat. Choose from the wide variety of Asian sauces to add flavour. Stir foods continuously to stop them sticking to the pan or wok.

- **Steam** – Steaming is a simple and very healthy way to prepare foods. You can cook food quickly with minimal nutrient loss, and add flavouring or seasonings to the water for extra taste.

- **Grill** – Small surfaces of the food are exposed to direct heat, allowing fat to drip away. You could use the grill of an oven, a BBQ or an indoor health grill.

Day 219 tip – Move more

Make like a fidget, and don't sit still

Do you know someone who always seems to have ants in their pants? It's more than likely they're lean because fidgeting has some proven weight-loss benefits. Scientists had volunteers avoid exercise, and eat an extra 4000 kilojoules a day for 8 weeks (about 10 chocolate biscuits). Some people gained 7kg, while others gained only 2kg. To help explain this, the subjects were outfitted with pedometers to measure their movement, and determine how much energy they expended each day. The difference appeared to be the fidget factor. The small weight-gainers didn't do extra exercise, but they moved more throughout the day. It was the small, fidgeting-like movements that separated the fast gainers from those who stayed slim. This could be standing up often, stretching, maintaining good posture, and just an inability to sit still. Another study found that fidgeting can burn off an extra 500 kilojoules (1200 calories) a day.

Living it

By moving more in everyday life, you can prevent weight gain. Even small amounts of movement all add up, and help to burn fat. Every muscle movement burns kilojoules and uses up some of the excess energy that might otherwise be stored as fat. This may help explain why some people gain weight easier than others.

Day 220 tip – Motivation and mindset

Use lists to help you lose

With time so precious, and our minds so preoccupied, lists can help to make sure you don't forget the important things. And you'll get a sense of satisfaction when you can cross things off. Write it down and make it happen. Put your lists on a piece of paper or use a variety of electronic equivalents like spreadsheets and email programs, PDA's and time management software.

Living it

Here are some practical ways you can use lists to help you get results.

- **To-do lists** – Once you have broken down your goals into mini-steps, add the tasks you need to complete onto your daily or weekly to-do list. You can also prioritise your list by ranking each task from the most important to least important.

- **Shopping lists** – Transfer the ingredients from the meals on your menu plan straight to your shopping list, and don't leave home without it. You'll then be much less likely to impulsively buy junk food.

- **Menu lists** – Make a list of the recipes you'd like to try in the future as you flick through magazines or recipe books. You can also create a list of your favourite, healthy recipes for breakfast, lunch, dinner and snacks.

Day 221 tip – Good food

Eat more fish and seafood

How often do you include fish in your diet? Nutrition research has clearly shown that your weight (and your heart) can benefit from eating fish and seafood regularly. The type of fat in fish – omega-3 fatty acid – can only be manufactured by your body in small amounts, so you need extra from your diet. All seafood contains varying amounts of omega-3 fatty acids, although deepsea fish tend to be the richest. Canned fish like sardines, salmon, herrings and tuna are also good sources of omega-3 fatty acids. Another benefit for weight loss is that fish has a fairly low fat and kilojoules content compared to other meats. For example, a 150 gram flathead fillet has 1.5 grams of fat, 150 grams of skinless chicken breast has 6 grams of fat, and 150 grams of lean beef (rib eye) has 8.5 grams of fat. Naturally, any benefits from eating seafood are reduced if it is battered, fried or covered in a butter or cream-based sauce.

Living it

Try to include at least two servings of fish or seafood every week, using low-fat cooking methods (grill, steam) and sauces (lemon juice, soy).

Day 222 tip – Move more

Follow these extra tips on interval training

Let's bring our focus back to the importance of interval training. By this stage in your program long, slow cardio just won't cut it. Intensity is the key! The puffing and red faces show it, the evidence I've seen with my clients proves it, and scientific research backs it up. An additional study on interval training showed that just 15 minutes of interval training over a two-week period was enough to improve exercise performance by almost 100%.

Living it

Imagine improving your exercise performance by 100% in just 2 weeks. That means you have a greater capacity to exercise, to burn extra kilojoules and use more fat as fuel. The study involved between four and seven 30-second bursts of 'all out' cycling followed by 4 minutes of recovery cycling between each interval on 3 days a week for 2 weeks. These subjects weren't even beginners, but they weren't doing intervals. More isn't necessarily better. If you can read a book or magazine while you're on an exercise bike, you are going too slowly. If you're not puffing at any stage of your walks, you're going too slow. Ignite your fat-burning potential with intervals.

Here are a few additional ideas on how you can incorporate interval training into your routine.

- Do 5 x 60-second intervals with 3 minutes of active recovery in between.
- Do 10 x 40-second bursts on a treadmill on maximum incline and 2 minutes of active recovery with no incline in between.
- Pyramid your intervals by doing 80 seconds, 60 seconds, 40 seconds, 20 seconds, 10 seconds with 3 minutes of active recovery in between.
- Do 2 or 3 interval cardio workouts a week alternating between days of longer, slower, steady state training.

- -

Day 223 tip – Motivation and mindset

Be your own fat loss coach

There are some basic tools that fat loss coaches use to help their clients get results. Try being your own coach. Who better to develop a good understanding of your strong and weak points; likes and dislikes?

Living it

Here are some of the tools and strategies that I use as a fat loss coach, so why not incorporate them into your own life. You'll find more information on many of these strategies throughout the book.

- Prioritise yourself.
- Have a non-weight related long-term goal.
- Set goals that focus on the process.
- Have an action plan to achieve your goals.
- Identify the barriers that are limiting your success.
- Learn from the past.
- Find ways to be accountable.
- Reward your successes along the way.
- Continually seek out new information and healthy recipes.

Day 224 tip – Good food

Make your supermarket a weight-loss helper, not a hindrance

The majority of foods people eat usually come from the supermarket. In other words, the choices you make as you walk through the supermarket isles will have a major impact on your body shape. A few minor changes in your shopping habits can make a big difference to your health and your weight.

Living it

Never go food shopping when you're hungry, or without a list. These strategies will also help you understand food labels, skip past the junk food isle and examine your shopping habits. Do you tend to come home with more than you intended? Do you plan your meals and shop with a list? Do you give in to the temptations at the checkout? Is your trolley loaded with lots of fruit and (especially) vegetables? What proportion of your food is highly processed and packaged? Do you experiment with different vegetables, spices and legumes? Be aware of and address any shopping habits that could be having a negative impact on your weight and your health.

Day 225 tip – Move more

Get in 'the zone' with your exercise

Why does an hour of training fly by for some but seem to drag on for others? According to one study, it can all come down to your exercise 'flow'. This term was first used by psychologists to describe artists who are deeply involved in their work, but it relates well to exercise. It's a feeling of being totally focused, in control and absorbed in what you're doing (like being in 'the zone'). It helps explain why some people stick with and enjoy a particular sport or exercise program while others drop out.

Living it

Finding your exercise 'flow' is a personal thing that's all about getting total absorbed in an activity and staying in the moment. If you can connect your thoughts, feelings and perceptions as you exercise, you'll be more likely to become a person who exercises for the fun of it and be motivated to exercise again and again so you can enjoy the pleasures and rewards you feel from it. Below are some ways to help you find your exercise flow.

- **Balance your skills with the activity** – Find an activity that's the right balance between comfort and challenge for you.

- **Have a clear goal** – Set goals that help you focus on the process, not the outcome. For example, focus on walking 7 kilometres in an hour, not on how much you weigh. This helps you concentrate on your actions and avoid distractions.

- **Tune in to how exercise makes you feel** – You are looking for the inner rewards of the activity itself. Being mindful and attentive of what you are doing, including your breathing and movement. These are the positive feelings that will make you choose to exercise not feel you have to do it.

- **Use variety** – Try different activities and exercises to compare the different levels of satisfaction you feel. You'll be more likely to find what suits you best.

Day 226 tip – Motivation and mindset

Embark on a do-it-yourself overhaul

If you have moved beyond the 'kinda-sorta-ready' phase and genuinely feel it's time to make some changes, you could try a do-it-yourself overhaul. If you want to transform your body shape, maybe there are some dramatic changes you could make that will help you get results. These are the types of things that are out of your comfort zone but could be just the trick to unleash your hidden potential.

Living it

If you are going to make a drastic change, you still need to focus on small, gradual steps, so only make one change at a time. Start by clearing out your food pantry and fridge of junk and restocking them with healthy food choices. You could also consider some of the more drastic changes people often make to turn things around, like hiring a personal trainer or signing up for boot camp. There are many additional ideas throughout this book that will help you step out of your comfort zone and overhaul your lifestyle.

Day 227 tip – Good food

Don't get behind bars. Breakfast cereal bars found guilty of health food fraud

Breakfast cereal bars are promoted as a quick and healthy breakfast alternative. While they often share the same name as the popular cereals, they are very different when it comes to nutritional value and kilojoule content. The bars are usually held together with a sticky mix of various sugars, which doubles their sugar content and halves the fibre content.

Some are also high in saturated fat and should really sit alongside the chocolates in the supermarket isle, not the breakfast cereals.

Living it

Don't assume breakfast cereal bars are a healthy alternative to a regular bowl of cereal with skim milk. Their high sugar content makes them a poor choice for weight control. Other quick breakfast ideas include a piece of fruit, raisin toast, a skim milk smoothie or reduced-fat yoghurt.

Day 228 tip – Move more

Forget about the fat-burning zone

The fat-burning zone is used as a guide on how hard to push yourself during exercise. You might see it displayed on cardiovascular exercise equipment or in the manual of a heart rate monitor. The fat-burning zone is given as a percentage of your maximum heart rate (220 minus your age) and is usually around 50–65%. This is a lower level than the cardiovascular zone (65%–85%), which is designed to boost your fitness. There is a lively debate in the fitness industry about what is the best heart rate zone to train in to maximise fat loss. According to scientific research, the lower fat-burning zone burns a high proportion of fat as fuel, but the higher intensity zone uses a greater total amount of kilojoules, and ultimately fat.

Living it

Don't get too concerned about all these zones. Lower heart rate zones are an ideal target for unfit beginners because the pace can be maintained over a longer period of time to help burn lots of kilojoules. As you get fitter, exercise at the highest intensity that is tolerable and safe, and burn maximal kilojoules in the time that you have.

Day 229 tip – Motivation and mindset

If you are in a relationship, get your partner involved

If your partner joins you along the path to better health, it will make the journey that much easier. You can motivate and encourage each other while moving together towards a common interest. Exercising with your partner can also help to keep you motivated. Why not go for a walk or bike ride together instead of planting yourself in front of the television. One study showed that 50% of married individuals who started an exercise program on their own dropped out, while 92% of couples were still with the program after 12 months. Lack of support from a partner is one of the main reasons people drop out of exercise programs. It's also helpful if you both eat the same foods. Placing one person on a different diet can make them feel isolated and increases food preparation, which will be difficult to maintain over the long-term.

Living it

The support and understanding that only a partner can give provides you both with a unique opportunity to work together towards a healthy, leaner future.

Day 230 tip – Good food

Indulge occasionally, but have a measure for 'occasionally'

I am all for indulging occasionally. You won't last long by completely depriving yourself of favourite foods and treats. You can still enjoy small portions of high-fat and high-kilojoule foods once in a while. And here's where things get a little grey. What does occasionally or once in a while actually mean? To me, it means once a week or once a fortnight. To my dear, sweet grandma – it means every day.

Living it

Having a treat is fine. It helps to know that you don't have to completely eliminate your favourite foods.

But think about how often you'll indulge. The first step is to indulge less than you are now. Then monitor your results and your treats. If you are happy with your results, there may be room for more regular treats. If you are not happy with your rate of weight and fat loss, cut back a little more. Over time, healthy eating will become a habit and you may not rely on treats as much.

Day 231 tip – Move more

Burn an extra 400 kilojoules (100 calories) a day

Losing body fat works best when you combine strategies that reduce your kilojoule intake with strategies that burn off extra fuel. Burning off an extra 400 kilojoules (100 calories) a day may not seem like much, but when you add it to your existing exercise routine, it really adds up.

Living it

Here are seven easy ways you could burn extra kilojoules each day. Adopt one today, or mix and match so you do at least one on each day of the week. These little changes won't even feel like exercise, but they are the long-term movement habits of someone who is lean. Why not adopt them yourself?

- **Wash the car** – Skip the drive-through and wash your vehicle on the weekend. Add a little polish and elbow grease, and your car and body will thank you for it.

- **Take the dog for a walk** – Just 20 minutes with the family pooch (or the neighbour's) is all it takes, and you could both probably do with the exercise.

- **Take the stairs** – Look to use the stairs every chance you get. You'll need to use a few to burn off 400 kilojoules, but you can add them up over the course of the day.

- **Play outside with the kids** – Enjoy a few games that involve running around. In 15 minutes you'll have used up 400 kilojoules and feel a lot better than if you had watched TV.

- **Cook dinner** – Spend 30 minutes in the kitchen: chopping and walking from the fridge, stove, sink and even the herb garden all adds up, and you'll have a healthy dinner to show for it.

- **Work in the garden** – Just 20 minutes of weeding, composting, fertilising and pottering will keep things looking good, and help you burn those 400 kilojoules.

- **Wash the dishes** – Give the dishwasher a break and volunteer yourself for some quality time with the pots and pans. Just 30 minutes should get the job done.

Day 232 tip – Motivation and mindset

Keep up to date with the latest in food, fitness and fat loss

Advice on health and lifestyle changes rapidly. Only a few years ago we used to talk about simple and complex carbohydrates, but the glycemic index blew that out of the water. Interval training and the importance of fish and seafood are also key weight-loss strategies that have only recently been recognised. It helps to stay up to date with any new information and research on health, fitness and weight control. Scientific studies are released almost daily that recommend new strategies, confirm old ones, and dispel myths and misunderstandings.

Living it

Knowledge is power – motivational power. Scan the Internet, read books and subscribe to magazines that motivate and educate. And you can subscribe to my free weekly email tip, the Better Body Update. See day 178 for details on how to subscribe.

Day 233 tip – Good food

Get creative, and make healthy foods taste great

Do you love celery sticks? Great if you do, but I don't. No matter how healthy something is, unless it tastes good it's pretty hard to stick with it over the long-term. Do you know anyone who has lasted more than a week or two on those 'eat nothing but soup' diets? I doubt it. Taste is the most common reason people choose the foods they do, and lack of taste is often reported as a deterrent when changing to a healthy diet. While cutting down your fat intake is important in reducing your kilojoule intake, you'll need to employ some tricks and special ingredients to keep things tasty.

Living it

Small amounts of sugar and fat are still needed to make a healthy diet palatable. For example, there is a place for small amounts of strong flavoured fatty foods, such as olive oil, nuts, avocado and parmesan cheese. Below are some other ways to add flavour to a healthy, lower fat diet.

- **Herbs and spices** – Use a wide variety of herbs and spices to liven up any meal.
- **Relish and pickles** – Add fat-free flavour to sandwiches and snacks.
- **Mustards** – American, English, French, German, wholegrain and Dijon all add lots of flavour.
- **Chili** – Use tobasco, chili powder, sweet chili, chili paste and fresh chili to all sorts of meals.
- **Marinades** – Can use a range of low-fat ingredients including white wine, red wine, sherry, garlic, ginger, lemon juice, soy sauce, hoi sin sauce and sweet chili sauce.

Day 234 tip – Move more

Choose your exercise equipment wisely

A great way to exercise in the comfort of your own home is with exercise equipment, including treadmills, steppers, rowers, bikes and elliptical striders. A recent study compared the kilojoule-burning potential of six different machines, and the results showed that for an equivalent level of perceived exertion (see day 63) the treadmill burned the most kilojoules. The more muscles a machine uses, the more kilojoules you'll burn.

Machine used with a 'somewhat strong' intensity	Kilojoules used per hour
Treadmill	2950
Stepper	2625
Cross-country ski machine	2590
Rower	2535
Cycle with moving handles	2130
Stationary bike	2084

Living it

While it appears that a treadmill is a good choice for exercise equipment, you will also have to weigh up factors like price, noise and space. The best piece of exercise equipment is one that you find easy and enjoyable to use.

Day 235 tip – Motivation and mindset

Help your family help you

Having the support of those closest to you'll play a big part in your ongoing motivation, and ultimately your success. It helps to have a network of people who can help you on your journey. But don't just hope that they'll know what to do, make it clear what you expect of them.

Living it

Make the following suggestions to your immediate family and let them help you in your journey.

- **Tell them why it's important** – Once your family members understand your perspective, and how much you value their help, they may be more likely to offer support.

- **One in, all in** – Different meals for different people makes food preparation and cooking very difficult. Explain how healthier eating can benefit everyone, and start off slowly to minimise any resentment at the change of routine.

- **Time sharing** – Keep a wall chart or calendar so you're family members know when you'll be exercising and give you space to work out in peace.

- **Don't use a lack of support as an excuse** – If you find it hard to get the support of your family and friends, seek the professional help of a personal trainer or dietician.

Day 236 tip – Good food

Be aware of your body's hunger signals (and stop eating when you're full)

One way to prevent overeating is to increase your awareness of your hunger and fullness levels. This can help to increase your awareness of three separate issues: eating without hunger, waiting too long to eat when you are hungry, and eating after you are full. No hunger eating is a problem for people who use food when they are bored or unhappy. Waiting until you're starving before you eat distorts your awareness of how much you need to feel full and can therefore trigger food binges. Finally, eating large portions and eating too quickly can result in a level of fullness that is higher than what your body needs.

Living it

Start to think about how hungry you are before you eat, and how full you feel when you are eating. This may take a conscious effort for a while, but it can help to moderate your kilojoule intake. You can also use the scale below to put a measure to how you feel. Try not to eat till you are around level 4 or 5, but don't let it drop to levels 1 or 2. Eat slowly and stop when you get to level 6.

1. As hungry as I have ever felt
2. Ravenous
3. Peckish
4. You're starting to feel like food, but not that hungry
5. You feel just right – neither hungry or full
6. Comfortably satisfied
7. You're full
8. Feeling very full
9. Stuffed, your stomach hurts a little
10. Sick, uncomfortable, difficult to move

Day 237 tip – Move more

Make the most of your exercise equipment

If you own a piece of exercise equipment, don't let it become an expensive clothes horse. Used effectively, exercise machines can add consistency to your exercise routine, and help to accelerate your results.

Living it

Here's how to get the most out of five of the most common exercise machines.

- **Treadmills** – To compensate for the lack of wind resistance, make sure the incline is at least 2–4%. Holding on to the handles also cuts your kilojoule use by a third, so only hold on when you need to.

- **Exercise bikes** – Try to vary your routine by using different levels of resistance and pedalling speeds. You can also stand on the pedals for some extra intensity. Bikes are also ideal for interval training.

- **Rowing machines** – Rowing should be about 60% legs and 40% arms, so really straighten your legs forcefully. Continually work on increasing your stroke rate per minute by measuring your time over a set distance.

- **Steppers** – Make sure you take deep, full steps and don't rest on your elbows. If you feel comfortable with the machine, try marching while moving your arms instead of holding on.

- **Elliptical trainers** – Really crank up the resistance on these machines, otherwise momentum tends to do most of the work for you. Try going backwards, crouching and using no hands for a little variety.

Day 238 tip – Motivation and mindset

Don't wait to be the next biggest loser

Reality TV shows about weight loss can create unrealistic expectations about a quick fix. While shows like the biggest loser and celebrity overhaul shows can be motivating, they also have the potential to be harmful. Following are some important points to consider.

1. Viewers watching might think that to achieve the same results they need to push themselves as hard as the contestants. But pushing untrained overweight or obese individuals to that extent without supervision is very dangerous, and could increase their risk of suffering a heart attack.

2. Contestants lose large amounts of weight quickly, which is unlikely to be sustainable over the long-term. Yet this creates an expectation of fast weight loss for the viewers. You don't have to train 6 hours a day to get results.

3. Using just weight as a measure of success is short sighted and unreliable. The focus should be on health, energy, wellness and how your clothes fit you, not on how much you weigh.

Living it

Television shows about weight loss are about entertainment not education. A longer-term approach to weight and fat loss is a better reality.

Day 239 tip – Good food

Realise that an apple a day is not enough, but it's close

Fruits are often grouped with vegetables, like the advice to eat 'seven servings of fruits and vegetables a day'. But fruit and vegetables are different and it's important to look at them separately. If you're eating too much fruit, you may find it hard to lose body fat. Like vegetables, fruit is packed with fibre and nutrients. But fruit is sweet because it's packed with sucrose, making it much higher in kilojoules than water-rich vegetables. Fruit is not an unhealthy food and it's a better choice than biscuits or chocolate, but it is high in kilojoules and you need to keep your portion sizes under control.

Living it

Where you should be aiming for 4–6 servings of water-rich vegetables a day, you should only have about two daily servings of fruit. Have fruit with your breakfast cereal, in skim milk smoothies or as a snack between meals. Try to keep your fruit intake under control and focus on ways to eat more water-rich vegetables.

Day 240 tip – Move more

Forget passive exercise machines

Passive exercise equipment is a type of machine you strap yourself into or strap onto yourself that makes your muscles move for you. There are large-scale machines that move your body, electronically powered exercise bikes, and other devices that make your muscles twitch. The concept is that you can get into shape while doing nothing except sitting around and watching TV. The reality is that these machines don't work no matter which celebrity provides testimonials, and some have even been banned because the advertising is misleading.

Living it

Whole gyms used to be based on this fallacy. Just remember the golden rule when it comes to passive exercise: 'if you don't do the work, it doesn't work'. If you aren't puffing, if your heart isn't beating faster, if you don't heat up a little, you are wasting your time. You need to generate heat to burn energy, and you won't burn off fuel if some powered gadget is doing the moving for you.

Day 241 tip – Motivation and mindset

Spend time with people who inspire you

Are there people in your life who seem to lift your mood and make you feel you can achieve anything? The more time you spend with people who have achieved what you want, the more their qualities and characteristics will rub off on you. Research has shown that modelling the behaviour, thoughts and attitudes of successful people can help a person become more successful. It creates the mindset of 'if they can do it, so can I'.

Living it

Pick someone you admire and ask yourself how can you emulate this person? Whenever you face a difficult situation, ask yourself how this person would act in this situation. What would this person do? What choices would they make, and are they suitable for you? Even if you don't have a weight-loss role model, resolve to spend more time with positive, optimistic people.

Day 242 tip – Good food

Be wary of artificially sweetened foods

Many dieters rely on artificial sweeteners to satisfy their sweet tooth with less kilojoules, but I question their health benefits over the long-term. It's best to eat foods close their natural state, making artificial sweeteners something to cut back on. Obviously, they help to reduce your kilojoule intake. One study revealed that people who replaced sugar-sweetened foods with aspartame-sweetened items, such as soft drinks, lowered their calorie intake by 7–15%. But research has also shown that people who know they're eating artificially sweetened foods tend to compensate by eating other high-fat foods. For example, drinking an artificially sweetened cup of tea with a biscuit, or a having a diet cola with a hamburger. Studies have also shown that aspartame increases the desire to eat in some people.

Living it

Watch the foods you eat with artificially sweetened products, especially the combination with junk foods such as a burger and diet cola. Use artificial sweeteners in moderation, as there is some uncertainty about their impact on your health over the long-term. It may also help to have a variety of different sweeteners to avoid having too much of the one type.

Day 243 tip – Move more

Eat enough iron to feel energetic enough to exercise

Iron is an important mineral for energy production, yet iron deficiency is extremely common in Australia, especially among women. A study on women showed that a low level of iron may impair body fat reduction. The iron deficient women generated less body heat, and were more likely to use glucose as fuel rather than body fat when placed in a cold environment. It seems that an iron deficiency slows down the metabolic rate, which may restrict fat use and total kilojoule expenditure. Symptoms of a low iron intake such as tiredness and fatigue can also influence your health, reducing your ability and motivation to exercise.

Living it

Eat lean red meat two or three times a week to make sure there is plenty of iron in your diet. If you feel you have any symptoms of iron deficiency (anaemia) such as lethargy, reduced ability to exercise, poor stamina and frequent infections, see your doctor for a blood test.

Day 244 tip – Motivation and mindset

Stress a little less

Stress is fattening, and it can make losing weight harder than it needs to be. From a physiological perspective, stress triggers the release of the hormone cortisol, which promotes fat storage. Cortisol tends to distribute fat deep inside your abdominal cavity and around your organs. This 'visceral' fat is the most dangerous to your health, and it helps to explain why stress contributes to poor health in everyone, no matter what your weight is. Stress also has an impact on your emotional health, increasing food cravings and fatigue. Feeling tired or stressed can also cause people to overeat in an attempt to boost their energy levels or find comfort.

Living it

Learning to better manage your stress will help you manage your weight. Everybody responds to stress management differently, just as they respond differently to stressful situations. Experiment with different strategies to determine what works best for you. In addition to learning relaxation techniques (which you'll find on day 277), here are some general strategies to help your body manage and prevent chronic stress:

- Eat well
- Exercise regularly

- Improve your time management skills
- Get enough sleep
- Take time to play and have fun
- Prioritise some time to do something you enjoy (time with family, gardening, fishing, etc.)
- Seek counselling if you are struggling to manage stress on your own.

Day 245 tip – Good food

Enjoy a hot breakfast once in a while (conditions apply)

There is hot breakfast, and there are fatty hot breakfasts. You can still enjoy a hearty feast, but there are some smarter choices you can make to prevent it 'sticking to your sides'.

Living it

When it comes to hot breakfasts, use the table below for some tasty yet healthier ideas to go for.

Instead of ...	Go for ...
Bacon	Lean bacon, low-fat ham, smoked salmon
Sausages	Grilled mushrooms, grilled tomatoes
Hash browns	Baked beans, steamed spinach
Fried eggs	Poached egg, hard-boiled egg (single portion)
Buttered toast	Multigrain bread, no butter or margarine
Scrambled eggs with full-cream milk	Scrambled 1 whole egg, 1 extra egg white and skim milk
Hollandaise sauce	Small portion, mustard, no sauce or tomato sauce

Day 246 tip – Move more

Going downhill has benefits as well

If you hate walking or running up hills, there is good news. A recent study found that while walking uphill was better for clearing fats from the blood, walking downhill reduced blood sugar more and improved glucose tolerance. It's not clear why the different types of exercise had different effects on fats and sugars in the blood, but the important thing is that both had benefits. The only negative is that downhill training puts extra pressure on the knees.

Living it

Walking downhill can be a good starting point if you have been inactive for some time. It's much easier, but will still be beneficial for weight control and kilojoule burning. The challenge will be to find a way to just go downhill without getting back to where you started (unless you live near a cable car). One option would be to walk down the stairs in a building, and use the elevator to go back up.

Day 247 tip – Motivation and mindset

Ditch the diet pills

The lure of easy weight loss is hard to resist. There are countless dietary aids, pills and powders available at supermarkets and pharmacies claiming to help you strip fat, speed up your metabolism and reduce your appetite. Yet there is no formal process to test the effectiveness of these products, and the claims are based on little or no scientific evidence. Even if they did work, you'd have to keep taking them forever to maintain any effects. These supplements can also have side effects and are associated with medical risks, just like prescription medication. Don't assume they are safe because they are 'natural'.

Living it

You might want to steer clear of the following additives.

- **Brindleberry** – You have to love a product made from the rind of an exotic fruit. Sounds great, does nothing.

- **Chitosan** – What a great way to make money out of leftover prawn and crab shells. Grind them up into a pill and flog them off as a weight-loss miracle cure.

- **Ephedra and synepherine** – The herb ephedra is a source of ephedrine, a powerful but deadly appetite suppressant that is banned in some countries. Supplement companies seeking to copy the effects of ephedrine without the side effects have been using synepherine, a citrus compound. But synepherine has been shown to elevate blood pressure.

- **Guarana** – Guarana is very similar to caffeine. No studies have reported on the effects of guarana on weight loss. Guarana can interact with drugs used to treat high blood pressure.

Day 248 tip – Good food

See biscuits for what they are – junk food

Biscuits might seem like an easy snack or a convenient addition to your cup of tea or coffee, but they are junk food, plain and simple. They are full of fat, sugar, salt and kilojoules, and are low in anything resembling nature or good nutrition. Some varieties have more fat and salt than potato crisps. They can also be high in trans fats, the worst kind for your heart, while some popular biscuits contain more sugar than flour. And don't be fooled by the 'healthy', low-fat alternatives. Most reduced-fat biscuits have extra sugar, so they still can have a similar (high) kilojoule content. Reduced-fat biscuits can still be frighteningly high in fat, which just highlights how bad the normal varieties are.

Living it

Try not to make biscuits an everyday food. Fruit is a far more nutritious snack, but just as sweet and convenient. Cracker breads can also give you that crunch with more fibre, and far less fat and kilojoules. It's one whole aisle in the supermarket you can breeze by.

Day 249 tip – Move more

Learn to love exercise

Have a look at the body of someone who loves to exercise and it's unlikely you'll see an overweight person. So what common characteristics do people who love exercise have, and how can you mimic them? You probably know that focusing on the distant benefits of exercise isn't the best motivation. It's the same for everyone. People who love exercise shift their focus from distant, external outcomes like losing weight to positive, internal experiences like how exercise makes them feel today. If you don't get something out of every single workout, you probably won't keep doing it.

Living it

Health and fitness is something other people enjoy, so there's no reason why you can't enjoy it too. If you have any negative thoughts about exercise, you might need to rethink your attitude. It may take a little time to start enjoying the feeling of movement if you have been inactive for a while. That's normal. Focus on the immediate benefits of exercise, like how you feel afterwards. If you can have a positive attitude and be patient, you'll be rewarded.

Day 250 tip – Motivation and mindset

Never, ever give up. Quitters never win

The most common mistake people make when they first begin to change their lifestyle is they quit. It takes time to decide to change, it takes time to progress, it takes time to generate momentum, and it takes time to see results. Many beginners don't allow themselves that time, and give up just when they are on the verge of making progress and overcoming the barriers that have held them back in the past.

Living it

The process of improving your health and your lifestyle takes patience and persistence. Get rid of that mentality that if you don't see fast or extensive results you give up. Make changes slowly so you don't feel like quitting. Give yourself 12 months, not 12 days. Expect slow change, and allow for it. Ask yourself why things will be different this time, and what it felt like when you quit in the past. Tell yourself that quitting is not an option, and move forward.

Day 251 tip – Good food

Limit your sugar intake

Being one of the top food additives in Australia doesn't make sugar a good choice, or a natural part of life as promoters would have you believe. Sugar is high in kilojoules and low in nutrients, and can bring your weight loss to a halt. Your body converts sugar into glucose thus triggering the release of insulin, which helps your body reduce the concentration of glucose in the blood (by storing it). However, insulin also triggers fat storage. It's better to supply your body with glucose from less processed sources, such as whole grains and vegetables, which are broken down slowly, used up as they go and reduce the need for insulin. The fibre in these foods is more likely to fill you up, and they also supply other important nutrients such as vitamins and minerals.

Living it

Sugar is concentrated in kilojoules and provides little fullness. Try to have it less often and in smaller quantities. Don't add sugar to foods, and watch out for hidden sugar in foods like biscuits, breakfast cereals and yoghurt.

Day 252 tip – Move more

Don't waste your time stretching before exercise

Regular stretching keeps your muscles flexible, but it's not necessary before you exercise. Research has shown that stretching before physical activity does nothing to prevent injury. Over 2500 people were divided into two groups, one who stretched before training and one who didn't. After performing over 50 hours of physical activity, there was no difference in injury rates. Some studies have actually shown that stretching before exercise can impair your performance.

Living it

Unless you have a history of injury, or are training at extremely intense levels, there is no need to stretch before you exercise. Performing a warm-up is still important, so do a gentle walk or slow run, and save your stretches till after your fat-burning workout.

Day 253 tip – Motivation and mindset

Don't let procrastination prevent your progress

If you keep putting off the moment when you will initiate changes to your eating and activity habits, your procrastination could be affecting your health. Don't just hope to get in better shape, or wait until you feel like it more than you do at the moment. There will never be the perfect time to start, so really, the best time to start is now.

Living it

Don't sabotage your own health and weight-loss goals. Why not make this weight-loss attempt different, and make it happen this time. In the long run, you know that making some changes will make you happy, and putting it off will make you sad, or annoyed at yourself. A good suggestion is to ask yourself the following questions when you notice yourself procrastinating.

- How important is the task I am putting off now?
- What are the advantages of starting right now?
- What are the disadvantages of leaving it until later?
- What am I wasting my time doing to avoid this task now?
- Will it kill me to do just a few minutes to get started?
- How can I break the task down into manageable chunks?
- What reward can I give myself for doing something/finishing it?
- Am I fed up with putting this off any longer?

Day 254 tip – Good food

If you have a sweet tooth, satisfy it with sweet foods not fatty foods

Do you have a sweet tooth, or is it really a fat tooth? The term sweet tooth is often used to explain cravings for sweet foods such as chocolates, cakes, biscuits, pastries, ice-cream and dessert. These foods are not only sweet they are all extremely high in fat. This presents the question: Is the sweet tooth just a fat tooth with a nicer name? Eating sweet foods actually increases your appetite for more sweet foods due to the roller-coaster effect they have on blood sugar. They can also increase your fat intake. A study found that people who have a sweet tooth eat 12 to 14 grams more fat a day than people without a sweet preference. Additional research has shown women are more likely to have a sweet tooth than men, especially as a source of comfort during periods of stress.

Living it

To see if your sweet tooth is really a fat tooth, try some sweet-only foods next time you have a craving. Foods like sorbet, jelly, boiled lollies, killer pythons, meringue and even fruit are all sweet but have virtually no fat. If your craving isn't satisfied after a sweet-only treat, you might be getting more kilojoules than you think. Over the long-term, cutting back on sugar and processed fats is an important step to improving your health.

Day 255 tip – Move more

Unleash your inner athlete

Most elite athletes are just like us and have to use hard work, determination and inspiration to reach the top. Fortunately, you don't have to be an Olympian to get great results. With most athletes following strict exercise and dietary programs, it can be the mindset that gives them that extra edge. Why not learn how they think, and apply their techniques to help give your weight loss a boost.

Living it

Here are some psychological strategies athletes use to improve their mental fitness, and boost their results.

- **Forget short cuts** – Stop trying to find some magic pill, miracle operation or magazine diet trick to help you get results. The answer lies within you. Others have achieved it and so can you, but you'll have to work at it.

- **Believe you can achieve** – According to the research, your belief in your own fitness ability is a primary factor in your success at sticking with your program. As your fitness improves, so will your confidence.

- **Prepare mentally** – Use visualisation and positive self-talk to build your confidence and self-belief.

- **Acknowledge your competition** – You may not be competing against an Olympian but you'll face challenges from other demands on your time like work, partners, travel time and social activities. Anticipate and prepare for them so they don't defeat you.

- **Set effective goals** – Set goals that are challenging, achievable, realistic and measurable. They need to drive you and light your internal fire. You also need to be accountable. Everyone knows what an athlete is trying to get better at. Create that type of pressure on yourself, and let people know what you are trying to achieve.

- **Cope with discomfort** – As your cardiovascular and interval training becomes more intense, you'll have to deal with some discomfort during training. That's part of the process, but make sure you build up gradually and focus on the rewards afterwards.

Day 256 tip – Motivation and mindset

Learn what 'not' to do from the average Aussie

When it comes to the battle of the bulge, it seems Australians have waved the white flag. The average Australian has put on more than 3 kilograms over the past 15 years, and we have some of the highest overweight and obesity rates in the world. Only around 15% of Australians are active enough to benefit their health. Studies also show that the average Australian consumes 112 grams of fat per day, which is more than double what is recommended to maintain a healthy diet, and nearly four times the daily amount recommended for fat loss. To get that much fat, the average Australian eats large portions and eats out too much. The five major sources of fat in the Australian diet are listed below.

Ranking	Source of fat	Grams per day
1. (44%)	Oils and fats (including butter, margarine and cooking oils)	50
2. (21.5%)	Meats/meat products	25
3. (19%)	Dairy foods (except butter)	21

Ranking	Source of fat	Grams per day
4. (5%)	Poultry	6
5. (10.5%)	Other (grains, eggs, nuts, seafood, fruit and vegetables)	10

Living it

Look to make changes that will have the most impact. Don't worry about the odd egg or handful of nuts. It's the butter, margarine, cooking oils, fatty meats and full-fat dairy products where you can generally make the most dramatic improvements.

Day 257 tip – Good food

Don't fool yourself that red wine is healthy

The suggestion that red wine is good for your health often interferes with the message about its weight gaining effects. While the antioxidants in red wine are beneficial for cardiovascular health, the same benefits can also be found from eating grapes or other fruits. For your heart, red wine is a reasonable choice among alcoholic beverages, but all alcohol will slow down weight loss. On the positive side, red wine is a fantastic, flavour-adding ingredient for recipes such as marinades, sauces and even soups. By using it in cooking, a good portion of the alcohol, and the kilojoules, will evaporate.

Living it

I don't want to be the no-fun police here. Red wine is an enjoyable part of life for many people (including myself) and can be included in moderation as part of a balanced lifestyle. Just don't kid yourself that drinking red wine is good for your health when you need to lose weight.

Day 258 tip – Move more

Spring clean to get lean (conditions apply)

Cleaning is a good way to boost your metabolic rate and burn kilojoules, but you need to do it with a little more vigor than normal to get any benefit. Housework on its own probably won't have significant benefits. A recent study found that people who engaged in at least one half-hour of heavy housework per week, such as vacuuming, washing windows and floors, were no less likely to be overweight than those who did no housework at all. But that doesn't stop you doing your housework with a little more gusto, or doing it on top of your regular exercise to accelerate your results. If you do your household chores for long enough, and with a little added intensity, it can burn 800–1000 kilojoules an hour, which is equivalent to a medium intensity aerobic workout.

Living it

Why not turn your cleaning into a kilojoule-burning workout? Sweeping, scrubbing, washing windows, mopping, vacuuming, washing and waxing the car, if performed a little bit faster than normal, can all get your heart rate up. Move quickly between jobs, and increase your level of movement around the house. Just don't rely on housework as your only form of exercise.

Day 259 tip – Motivation and mindset

Be aware of the critical life periods for weight control

Weight loss can be tough, but in combination with other life challenges it becomes even tougher. These difficult times have been identified as the critical periods or stages of weight control that could make or break your success, and include the following:

- after retirement from sport
- grief or bereavement
- redundancy or changing of jobs
- divorce or separation
- pregnancy
- marriage
- middle age for men (40 onwards), menopause for women
- during prolonged social/festive occasions
- after quitting smoking.

Living it

Challenges and setbacks are a part of life. But it's how you bounce back from these obstacles that can make a world of difference. This is not meant to downplay the significance of these critical periods, but to focus on the importance of not giving up completely. Adjust your plans; don't abandon them. Then when you begin to move on from these critical life periods you'll be in a better position to get back on track.

Day 260 tip – Good food

Eat more low-fat spicy foods

Would you like to raise your metabolism with some basic ingredients that are probably already in your pantry? Hot and spicy foods can boost your metabolism and help your body burn more kilojoules by elevating your body temperature and increasing your heart rate. They can also help with weight control by adding a unique fire and richness to foods that makes you want to eat smaller portions. The key ingredient is a substance called capsaicin, which is present in varying amounts in a number of spicy foods.

Living it

Spicy foods have the most benefit to your metabolism if they are consumed as a regular part of the diet, or at least three times per week. Look for ways to include more curry powder, cayenne peppers, chili powder, tobasco sauce, ginger, horseradish, wasabi and hot English mustard in your meals. They also need to be consumed as part of a low-fat diet, otherwise the extra energy from fat (such as coconut cream or a butter-based sauce) will counteract any benefit.

Day 261 tip – Move more

Forget about food combining. Try combining healthy eating with regular exercise

Have you heard that you shouldn't eat carbohydrates and protein together? There's absolutely no scientific evidence to support this claim. Most foods contain a combination of carbohydrates, protein and fat, and these nutrients are not designed to be separated. If you consider the fact that breast milk is designed for human infants, and that it contains a combination of all nutrients, this myth should be laid to rest. Your body secretes a variety of digestive enzymes quite capable of breaking down any food or combination of ingredients (even when we're infants). We also know that your body absorbs more vitamins and minerals when your diet is made up of a wide mixture of different foods. This type of diet gimmick, and the manipulation of nutritional facts, is used to sell diet books and programs. Unfortunately, people are drawn to them because it offers a weight-loss solution that is new and different, and doesn't involve exercise.

Living it

There is no justifiable reason to separate certain foods from others to boost weight loss. Don't let these types of wild claims distract you from the proven and most effective course of action – healthy eating and regular exercise.

Day 262 tip – Motivation and mindset

Know when to take the next step when your eating is out of control

If you've identified yourself as an emotional eater, and don't seem to be able to overcome it, there is help available.

You may require specialist treatment from a psychologist who specialises in food and weight control. Other eating disorders and conditions that may also benefit from treatment include food addiction, bulimia, disordered eating and excessive night-time eating. For some people, therapy is an important step on the road to recovery, helping you to change the way you think before changing the way you eat.

Living it

Here's how to know when it may be best to seek extra help with your eating:

- When you feel you have exhausted your knowledge and skills
- You are having difficulty understanding why you overeat
- You are having trouble separating yourself from some foods emotionally
- You find that making dietary changes makes things worse (e.g. more bingeing)
- You use laxatives and vomiting to control your weight
- You have a history of eating disorders
- Friends let you know they are worried about your eating habits.

Day 263 tip – Good food

Figure out your food triggers

Is there a pattern to your diet where certain people, places or thoughts trigger you to overeat? Some general eating triggers include emotions, locations and relations, and they can be brought on by internal sensations like blood sugar levels or external stimuli like the smell of a food. Other examples of food triggers include the time of day, watching TV, stress or being with certain friends, and they often have little to do with hunger or appetite. This is all part of the important process of identifying what causes you to overeat, and possibly why you have excess body fat.

Living it

Be on the lookout for situations that trigger your diet downfalls, perhaps with a food journal. It may help you to recognise the people or places that cause the most problems, allowing you to develop strategies to deal with them. For example, if you find yourself snacking on crisps while watching TV, try to watch less TV, or don't have crisps in the house.

Day 264 tip – Move more

Use gardening to help burn fat (conditions apply)

Gardening provides a wide variety of movements that have the potential to tone and strengthen your muscles, and burn some kilojoules. The more muscles involved in your activity, the more kilojoules you'll burn. In other words, 5 minutes of pruning will not exactly transform your body. Because gardening is a stop-start activity, it needs to be carried out for a long duration to help assist fat burning.

Living it

If you combine a range of vigorous and active movements such as digging, raking, pulling, walking and squatting, you can get a good, whole-body workout. While not a good substitute for cardiovascular exercise, it is an excellent addition to your exercise routine. Perform all movements at an energetic pace for maximum results.

Day 265 tip – Motivation and mindset

Boost your energy levels to boost your results

If you are tired and lethargic all the time, it's going to be hard to motivate yourself to exercise. On the other hand, feeling energetic can make you want to run faster, exercise more vigorously and continue your activity for longer.

Living it

Consider the following ways to add energy and vitality to your life.

- **Go for carb quality** – Low GI carbohydrates found in beans, wholegrain pasta, oats and vegetables digest slowly, giving you a gradual release of glucose into the blood stream and providing long-term energy.

- **Get enough sleep** – Fatigue may simply be due to a lack of sleep. It's going to be a lot easier to get yourself up and moving after a good night's rest. See day 169 for more on how to sleep better.

- **Get hydrated** – Many people fail to replace the 6–8 glasses of water they lose every day. Fatigue is a symptom of dehydration, so drink more water.

- **Vitamins and minerals** – Low levels of iron, and not getting enough nutrients from your food, can deplete you of energy.

- **Cut back on alcohol** – Alcohol is dehydrating and depletes your body of nutrients. Aim to have 3–5 alcohol-free days a week.

- **Manage your stress** – Over scheduling can be a major cause of fatigue. If you can't avoid being busy and rushed, try to at least compensate by scheduling some time to relax.

- **Rest and recreation** – Do something different regularly like seeing a show or visiting a new place. You may even enjoy a holiday to recharge the batteries.

Day 266 tip – Good food

Have eggs on the menu (conditions apply)

There seems to be a lot of conflicting advice about eggs, which have to be one of the most debated topics in nutrition. From a weight-loss perspective, egg whites are on par with water-rich vegetables and legumes as the ideal fat loss food. The yolk is a little high in cholesterol and fat, although it's a better choice than the fats found in butter, ice-cream and fast foods. One egg yolk contains around 5 grams of fat, with only 1.5 grams of saturated fat. Egg whites contain no fat. A recent study showed that having an egg for breakfast is one of the more filling choices you can make. Subjects who ate eggs felt fuller after breakfast and stayed fuller longer than those who ate a bagel. Although the kilojoule content of both meals was the same, the egg group ate 2400 kilojoules at lunch, compared with 3050 kilojoules by the bagel group. That's a massive 29% less kilojoules. The egg eaters also ate less total kilojoules over the day. Because of their high protein content, eggs have a much greater capacity to fill you up than breakfast cereal or bread.

Living it

Have an egg for breakfast, but try to have at least two or three whites and one yolk. Watch the high-fat company that eggs keep like butter, white bread, sausages, bacon, hollandaise sauce and hash browns.

Day 267 tip – Move more

Get a strong core to support your weight-loss efforts

Your 'core' is a generalised term used to describe a group of deep muscles in your abdomen, back and pelvic region. A strong core will help with fat loss, although more through association. It helps to improve your performance in all activities, making any exercise safer and more efficient. Strengthening your core will also better prepare you for resistance training, another vital tool you can use to promote fat loss. In addition, a stronger core can have a positive effect on your physical appearance, reducing the size of a flabby lower belly. This can boost your self-esteem and confidence. Finally, preventing back problems and developing your strength and balance will increase your opportunities, and desire, to be active and burn body fat.

Living it

To train and strengthen your core you need to consciously contract your abdominal muscles, sucking your belly button into your spine. This is called 'activating' your core and is something that may take a little time to get used to. Start out by activating your core muscles while stationary then gradually incorporate core activation into a variety of movements. There are plenty of books, DVDs and exercise classes designed to help you improve core strength. Over time, core activation will become a habit, especially during movements that place stress on your back.

Day 268 tip – Motivation and mindset

Be cool – It will help you burn more fat

The body seems to use more kilojoules to maintain body heat when you are cold, compared to the kilojoules it uses to cool itself when you are warm. This is because the body's system for cooling (sweating) is passive and requires no extra use of kilojoules, while cold temperatures stimulate an increase in metabolic rate and other kilojoule-burning responses such as shivering. This was emphasised in a study on the weight of two groups of soldiers who had identical rations and exercise programs, where those living in a cold climate lost more weight than the soldiers with the same lifestyle in a warm climate. Another study showed that a 5-degree drop in temperature increased metabolic rate by 10%. This also further dispels the myth of outdated weight-loss methods such as saunas, or exercising in three tracksuits and special suits to help you sweat off fat. These methods look good on the scales because they dehydrate you, but you would actually lose more fat (not water) by spending time in a cool room.

Living it

Practically speaking, don't start off your exercise in heavy clothing. Be a little bit cold when you start your workout. It won't take you long to heat up, and you'll burn more kilojoules overall. It will also be beneficial to avoid overheating in everyday life, such as overdressing and excessive use of heating in your car, home or workplace. It's not about being uncomfortably cold, but keeping a little cooler will help you burn more kilojoules.

Day 269 tip – Good food

Find peace with chocolate

Is the thought of life without chocolate unbearable for you? Chocolate is a powerful food, containing drug-like substances that alter your mood and your brain chemistry by acting like a stimulant, and an anti-depressant. There's no doubt it tastes great; over 50% of food cravings are thought to be centred on chocolate. Women especially are known to have a strong craving for chocolate, especially just before their period. Some people even confess to being addicted. What's more, the dark variety is a good source of antioxidants. The other reality is that all varieties are high in fat and kilojoules, and you can't eat large quantities of chocolate if you are serious about losing body fat.

Living it

Chocolate can still be enjoyed without guilt if you manage your portions. Savour a small amount to keep your cravings at bay. Portion-controlled servings, such as individually wrapped chocolate, may be particularly helpful. You can also try healthier choices like diet hot chocolate drinks, a chocolate-covered muesli bar or a hazelnut/chocolate spread on toast.

Day 270 tip – Move more

Don't let delaying tactics bring your results to a halt

Go to any gym, or watch people exercise anywhere, and you'll see some amazing delaying tactics. Take your pick between sitting around, daydreaming, resting between sets or machines, chatting, leaning on a machine, taking a long time to get a drink of water, fiddling with shoe laces. When you invest your time in exercise, why not make your workouts as effective as possible?

Living it

Is a lack of intensity in your training holding you back from getting results? When you exercise, ask yourself what percentage of time you are actually training at the right intensity, and not just visiting. Strive to beat your personal best times, weights, distances and efforts. From great effort comes great reward.

Day 271 tip – Motivation and mindset

Measure your waist-to-hip ratio

Waist-to hip-ratio measures the difference between your waist and your hip circumference. An uneven distribution of fat between the abdomen and the hips is a strong predictor of potential health problems. Waist-to-hip ratio is also a good way to assess the dangerous visceral fat stored around your internal organs. This is also a good time to compare the change in your waist circumference since you last measured it on day 19. Ideally, it's been 3–6 months since you last measured your waist, so hopefully you are progressing well.

Living it

To calculate waist-to-hip ratio, follow these steps.

1. Using a tape, measure your waist at the belly button and the hips at the widest point. Write down your measurements below:

    Waist _____ (in centimetres)   Hips _____ (in centimetres)

2. Divide the waist measurement by the hip measurement. This is your waist-to-hip ratio, which you can record here _____.

For example, someone with a 95cm waist, and a 100cm hip circumference has a waist-to-hip ratio of 0.95. There is a significantly increased health risks for insulin resistance, type 2 diabetes and high blood pressure if the ratio is greater than 0.95 for men and 0.8 for women.

Day 272 tip – Good food

Don't rely on the heart tick alone to select foods

The Heart Foundation's tick of approval can be seen everywhere, from fast food restaurants to the margarine aisle of your supermarket. The tick is designed to direct you towards better choices among specific categories of food. For example, a cheese with the Heart Foundation tick means that this is a good choice among cheeses for your heart. While this is beneficial for heart health, there may be better choices for your waistline. Healthy heart choices that are lower in saturated fat and salt can still be high in other fats or sugars. What's more, food manufacturers pay for the heart tick, so in some cases foods without the tick may be a better choice.

Living it

Don't rely on the heart tick alone when selecting foods. Use the nutrition information panel on food labels to compare the amount of kilojoules, fat, sugar, sodium and dietary fibre of a food. This will give you a more balanced view of the best choice for losing weight and body fat.

Day 273 tip – Move more

Get some new workout gear

It's a great feeling to put on some new exercise gear for the first time and go for a workout. Why not invest in a new pair of exercise shoes or workout clothes that fit you well, and make you feel good about yourself. You could even accessorise with an mp3 player, water bottle, pedometer, heart rate monitor, audio program or workout DVD. Having something new can inject some enthusiasm back into your exercise routine.

Living it

Look for a way to reward yourself with some new exercise gear. Why not link it to an exercise challenge, like training every day for a fortnight or beating a long standing personal best time or distance goal. You'll enjoy your new stuff even more knowing how hard you worked to earn it. Gradually get rid of any sloppy workout T-shirts as your body shape changes, and assure yourself you won't need them anymore.

Day 274 tip – Motivation and mindset

Revisit and revise your goals

As much as I'd like you to stay focused on the process and not the results, it's time to see if the process is actually working. After re-measuring your abdominal girth to calculate your waist-to-hip ratio, let's take stock and see how you're going.

Living it

Take your original waist measurement (day 19) and subtract your current waist measurement (day 271). Then divide this number by the original measurement and multiply by 100. For example, a person with a 103cm waist 6 months ago now has a 95cm waist. So 103 minus 95 equals 8. Then divide 8 by 103 to get 0.077. Now, multiply 0.077 by 100 to get the percentage of waist lost. In this case, it's 7.7%. Depending on your results, see the suggestions below to persist or reinvent your goals.

- **If you've lost more than 5% off your waist** – Well done, the changes you've made are working and your health has improved. The lifestyle you're living is getting you closer to your long-term goal. This could be a good time to give yourself a reward for your achievements so far.

- **If you've stayed the same or lost less than 5%** – Something's not working, so it may help to flick back through the book to find any problem areas. Don't punish yourself or give in. Revise your goals and focus on the areas that are holding you back. If you have been following all the principles in this book and have not seen significant results after at least 3 months, it may be advisable to see a doctor about any medical reasons that could be preventing weight loss.

Day 275 tip – Good food

Consider meal replacement shakes and bars (conditions apply)

I was surprised to read a study showing that there are some weight-loss benefits from using meal replacement drinks and bars. I have always thought these were a short-term solution, and therefore flawed. But the study was long-term and the improvements in food technology mean that these products can fill you up while also tasting good enough to be something you don't mind having regularly.

Living it

If you are juggling a hectic life, or have trouble exercising due to excess weight, meal replacements may be an option for you. They are obviously a better choice than junk food or takeaway. Speak to your doctor, pharmacist, nutritionist or fat loss coach first. Following are some guidelines on how to use meal replacements safely and effectively.

- Use meal replacements at the meals that cause you the most trouble. For example, if you already eat a healthy breakfast, focus on replacing lunch or dinner.

- Don't use a meal replacement for more than two meals a day.

- Over time, mix and match the meals you replace to maintain interest.

- As you begin to lose weight, rely less on meal replacements.

- Don't use meal replacements as a green light to eat junk at your other meals. Make your normal meals healthy to maximise your results.

- Avoid the cheap supermarket brands that are virtually all sugar and skim milk powder.

- If you get hungry, eat fruit between meals for added fibre.
- Don't forget to exercise as well.

Day 276 tip – Move more

If you're struggling for motivation, hire a personal trainer

An appointment with a personal trainer adds to your commitment to exercise, and can really help encourage and motivate you. Personal trainers give you individual attention and structure exercise programs around your specific needs. This not only increases the safety aspect, it increases your likelihood of getting results. Prices vary dramatically depending on the duration of your session, the quality of the trainer, if you are prepared to share your session, how many sessions you do a week, and how many sessions you pay for in advance.

Living it

If you are considering hiring a personal trainer, look into their qualifications, experience, availability, prices and packages, insurance, training location and registration with a fitness industry association. Better still, speak to the trainer's clients, and ask about their results. If price is a concern, even one shared half-hour session per fortnight could help keep you on track for around $20.

Day 277 tip – Motivation and mindset

Use relaxation techniques to prevent stress

Relaxation refers to a break from work or activity where the focus is on rest or pleasant recreation. It is still an alert state of mind, but it allows the body to let go voluntarily and helps to release tension. Relaxation can help to minimise the harmful effects of stress because it helps to reduce your heart rate, blood pressure, breathing rate, muscle tension, sweating, arousal and adrenalin level. There are many relaxation techniques you can use. Some are mainly physical, some are mental and some a combination of both. Depending on your preferences and how you feel, different techniques can be used.

Living it

Relaxation is different things to different people, but it may include having a bath, a massage, doing Tai Chi or listening to music. Below is a relaxation technique that uses breathing awareness, and it should only take a minute or two. Before you commence, make sure you are comfortable, in a place free from sudden sounds and interruptions, and where you can close your eyes and in be peace.

- Sitting or lying comfortably, close your eyes, and count backwards from 10 to 0.
- Using deep breaths, count slowly and say each number in your mind while exhaling.
- Allow several seconds to pass between numbers.
- After zero is reached, enjoy the relaxation before returning to an alert but relaxed state when ready.

Day 278 tip – Good food

Eat as many foods as you can that don't have a food label

Are most of your foods out of a packet? Mother Nature has blessed us with an incredible variety of foods to choose from. Why not try to eat more plant foods and experiment with new colours, flavours, aromas and textures in your diet? Plant-based foods such as vegetables, fruits, nuts, herbs, whole grains and legumes are less processed, so they are high in fibre and have a high ratio of nutrients to kilojoules. This slows down their absorption rate, helping to satisfy your hunger with less kilojoules and lose weight. Packaging, processing, powdering and preserving foods reduces their nutritional value. Artificial foods often include refined ingredients such as salt, sugar and chemically altered fats. When the ingredient list includes a bunch of numbers and chemicals you can't pronounce, there are probably better food choices you could make.

Living it

Try to eat more unprocessed plant-based foods, and be wary when you are pouring something out of a box, opening a packet or reconstituting something with water.

Day 279 tip – Move more

Play games that burn fat. Try some exer-tainment

One of the latest trends in health and fitness is exer-tainment or exer-gaming, which is the marriage of physical activity with video gaming. Designed for both children and adults, there is an increasing range of video games and exercise machines that almost 'trick' you into being active. One example is an exercise bike that's connected to a TV screen and the faster you pedal, the further you progress in a computer-generated race. When you go up hills on the screen, the resistance automatically increases, while it gets easier when you go down hills. Another more affordable option is a $100 game that connects to a PlayStation console and comes with miniature dance floor containing optical sensors. Players tap their feet to the correct pattern on the floor pad, based on cues on the screen. Another game uses a camera to monitor your movements and superimposes them on the screen, so you can compete in activities like boxing, dancing, baseball, tennis or jumping over rolling barrels.

Living it

It's unlikely that these games will be enough to help you lose weight on their own, but it's a fun way to spend your leisure time being active rather than sitting on the couch.

Day 280 tip – Motivation and mindset

Focus on what you gain, not what you lose

Most diets and infomercials get caught up in weight loss, fat loss, loss of centimetres and loss of a dress size. That may be what people want to hear, but it's so much more rewarding to shift your focus on what you have to gain through improving your health, eating better and moving more. You body is like an engine and if you can fine tune it and run it on good quality fuel, your performance will no doubt improve.

Living it

Have a measure of your success that doesn't involve weight loss. Being lean is vital for good health, but just as important is how you achieve this. Recognise the rewards that eating better and moving more have to offer. As you work towards losing body fat, try to focus on how you feel, your new energy levels, reduced stress levels, how well you sleep, and how you breathe easier during activity.

Day 281 tip – Good food

Only have a 'junk day' if you really need it

Some diets advocate a 'junk day' (also known as cheat day), where you strategically 'blow' your healthy eating plan. This is said to jump-start your metabolism, preventing your body from adapting to a lower kilojoule intake. But there's no real scientific evidence to back this up. Some people feel they need a junk day to keep their sanity and prevent cravings or binges throughout the week. But any food can be enjoyed in moderation as part of a healthy eating plan. It's better to have a more positive attitude towards healthy eating and seek out healthy recipes that taste great.

Living it

Only 'cheat' if you feel it's emotionally necessary, and not because you feel like it's going to help you lose weight. The benefits from a cheat day are probably more psychological rather than physical, especially during the early stages of improving your diet. Try to aim for a junk meal rather than a junk day.

Day 282 tip – Move more

Carry a weight while you walk (conditions apply)

Carrying extra weight while you walk adds variety and increases the demands on your heart and muscles, helping you to burn more kilojoules over a given distance. This weight can be in the form of dumbbells, a weight belt, a weighted vest, back pack or ankle weights. Research has shown that extra weight can increase your heart rate by 2–5%, which leads to a slightly higher level of conditioning and fuel burning, with no increase in speed.

Living it

Walking with dumbbells can cause shoulder problems in some people, while ankle weights should be avoided completely, as they can alter your balance. The best choice is a tight-fitting vest or backpack will help you burn extra kilojoules without altering your posture or placing stress on your joints. Another way to add a little extra weight on your long walks is a camelback water bladder, which adds 3 kilograms and keeps you hydrated.

Day 283 tip – Motivation and mindset

Make peace with your body

Very few people are totally satisfied with the way they look. There is nothing wrong with realising that you need to lose weight, but there are degrees of dissatisfaction. There is a strong relationship between body image and self-esteem. When your self-esteem is down, it's common to become preoccupied with negative thoughts about your weight, which can lead to comfort eating. Few of us have the genetics and body type to be on the cover of a magazine, but everyone can take action to improve their health. You can protect your self-esteem by focusing on self-improvement and self-acceptance.

Living it

Work on what you can change and accept what you can't. Don't judge your self-worth on your appearance, or aspire to unrealistic ideals that are airbrushed or surgically enhanced. Instead of wasting time and energy focusing on your imperfections, give yourself credit for eating better, exercising more and doing something positive for yourself. Losing weight and improving your health will boost your self-esteem, and you'll feel a greater sense of power and personal control, feel and perform better and be more likely to stay motivated. If you have more serious issues with your body image, it may help to seek professional counselling.

Day 284 tip – Good food

Eat nuts – small portions make for a great snack

Are you nuts about nuts? Their high fat and kilojoule content has made them a bit of a dietary danger zone, but that doesn't have to be the case. A recent study of people on a low-kilojoule diet showed that nuts can actually help with weight loss, making you feel full with their high protein and fibre content. They are indeed high in fat, but it's the good type – the mono-unsaturated fats – which are metabolised quickly and are good for your heart. You should have some fat in your diet, even when you are trying to lose weight and fat, making nuts a good snack choice and a tasty addition to salads.

Living it

All nuts have benefits, so a mixture is best. A rough guide is a small handful, or 30 grams a day. But make sure you consider how many other fats (healthy or otherwise) are in your diet. Their weight-loss benefit comes from including them (salt free) as part of low-kilojoule diet. Eat too many and they could bring your weight loss to a halt.

Day 285 tip – Move more

Leave the sports drinks for the marathon runners

Sports drinks are of no benefit if your training goal is weight loss. In fact they can hold back your results. Like fruit juice, soft drinks and cordial, sports drinks are just excess kilojoules that your body will have to burn off first before it can tap into stored body fat. Don't undo all your hard work in burning off kilojoules by adding them straight back on again. If you've heard different advice, that's because this is the opposite to what is recommended for athletes and people who are training very intensely for a long duration.

Living it

Sports drinks make it harder for you to lose body fat. Water is a better choice before, during and after exercise, unless you train intensely for an hour or more.

Day 286 tip – Motivation and mindset

Seeing is achieving – practise visualisation

Visual images can be a powerful motivating force, and you can use this to your advantage to help you lose weight. Using positive imagery is something athletes use to help them achieve success, such as imagining being first to reach the finish line. Seeing is believing because what we see can determine how we act. Imagining something you want to achieve over and over again puts your subconscious mind to work. Once you write something down or see a picture of your goal, your brain starts to work on that goal without you even realising it. This connection between picture and motivation only grows stronger as you achieve and see results.

Living it

Practising visualisation might seem a little strange, but what have you got to lose? You could imagine what your body will look like after you've lost weight or how it will feel when you complete your first fun run. By using positive imagery, and surrounding yourself with visual cues, you have a better chance of meeting your goals. So write down your goals, stick positive pictures on the fridge, tape an inspiring message to your computer, and think about what you want to achieve before going to sleep each night. In time, success will transfer from what your mind sees to reality.

Day 287 tip – Good food

Go vegetarian once in a while

One of the best ways to increase your vegetable intake, and reduce your kilojoule consumption, is to have vegetarian meals. Research has shown that a diet low in animal products and fat can help with weight loss. In one study, subjects on a vegan diet lost nearly double the amount of weight as a low-cholesterol diet group over a 14-week period; the vegetarian group also had a slightly elevated metabolism and improved sensitivity to insulin.

Living it

You don't need to be a permanent vegetarian to enjoy some of the benefits on offer. Seek out recipes for meals based on vegetables, whole grains and legumes, and try to have a vegetarian lunch or dinner at least once a week. Avoid the high-kilojoule, non-meat items like full-fat milk, butter, cream, cheese, eggs yolks, vegetable oil and full-fat yoghurt. It's also important to manage your portion size of nuts and seeds, avocados and starchy vegetables.

Day 288 tip – Move more

Use an mp3 player to make the most of your exercise

There's no shortage of gadgets and workout toys to make your exercise more interesting, but few can match the features of an mp3 player. They are lightweight, reasonably priced and can store hundreds if not thousands of songs on a device not much bigger than a box of matches. If you like to exercise alone, an mp3 player is a great addition to your training program.

Living it

Load your mp3 player with lots of songs that inspire you to go fast and hard, and make you want to get out there. You could also add some slower, more relaxing music for your cool down or a long relaxing stroll. Another great way to use your mp3 player is with podcasting. Download radio interviews, audio books or information programs. Have a look in the back of this book for more information on my 'Secrets of the diet whisperer' CD.

Day 289 tip – Motivation and mindset

Learn from our lean, Stone Age ancestors

For millions of years, humans lived as hunter-gatherers. Studies show these people were lean, muscular and relatively free of disease. A few thousand years ago we developed agriculture to help us stay in one area; instead of living a nomadic hunting lifestyle, people could settle down in one area and get their food from farming, including grain and dairy foods. But the onset of this new lifestyle has resulted in the evolution of a number of diseases of affluence, such as cancer, osteoporosis, diabetes and our current obesity epidemic.

Living it

For optimal health, and within reason, we need to find ways to eat and exercise like our genetic cousins from the Stone Age. Here are some practical examples:

- Buy leans cuts of meat
- Cook in healthy oils

- Cut back on processed grain foods
- Cut back on full-fat dairy products
- Eat a variety of different foods throughout the week
- Eat a variety of seasonal fruits and vegetables
- Be active by incorporating long walks, short sprints, lifting weights and dancing.

Day 290 tip – Good food

Have a garden salad, with a meal chaser

A recent study discovered that eating a broth-based soup or a low-kilojoule salad before a meal helps to significant reduce your kilojoule intake. Subjects who had a salad before their meal ate 12% fewer kilojoules overall than people who did not start with a salad. Because you're full at the start of a meal, you eat less later. It's also thought that the salad-eaters more than likely stop eating their main course earlier than they would otherwise because they believe they have eaten a lot of food. Salads also require a lot of chewing, adding time to the meal and again reinforcing the idea they have eaten enough. Researchers also discovered that a high-kilojoule salad containing a high-kilojoule dressing and cheese had the opposite effect, where subjects ate 17% more kilojoules more during the entire meal than if they did not eat a salad before. It was noted that a small amount of fat was helpful in the salad because it helps the body to absorb important nutrients.

Living it

Why not try a small garden salad with a glass of cold water just before your next lunch or dinner, and see how it affects you.

Day 291 tip – Move more

Don't let anything hold you back. Try something new

As we get older, fear becomes more dominant during our decision-making. We have more worries and responsibilities, and more things to weigh up when faced with risk-taking choices. There is even research to show that part of the brain develops to regulate our impulsive risk-taking behaviour as we age, especially in women. People become a prisoner to their comfort zone instead of taking a risk. To break this pattern and achieve more than you have in the past, you'll have to push the boundaries of your comfort zone.

Living it

Over the coming series of 'move more' tips, I will outline a variety of activity suggestions for you to try. By now you've hopefully built up a solid exercise routine of planned, cardiovascular exercise, and maybe even a little strength training each week. These different types of activities aren't necessarily the perfect fat-burning activities, but they add fun, adventure and something new. There's no need to worry about heart rate or puffing, just get out there and try something new. These are the type of activities that open up to you now that you are healthier, stronger and leaner. You might try just one of them, or all of them, and maybe even adopt one as a permanent addition to your routine.

Day 292 tip – Motivation and mindset

If you need a little extra motivation, try group support

Group programs for weight loss can add a different level of motivation and support, especially through the more challenging early stages. One study showed that participants assigned to a weight-loss support group, with weekly weigh ins, were nearly four times more likely to lose weight than those assigned to self-help. According to the study, the strongest motivation and support came from people who have been there themselves and succeeded. Bonds are formed and members help each other. The social aspect of group weight-loss therapy work tends to be popular with women, while men can still benefit from group exercise squads and gatherings.

Living it

There are a whole range of group options that you could investigate in your local area, including weight-loss meetings, healthy cooking classes or group exercise sessions in jogging, cycling, aquarobics or walking.

If there are none in your area, why not start your own. Exercising in a group is also ideal if you can only exercise in the dark, giving you safety in numbers. You could even try weight-loss online chat rooms and blogs to provide online support in the comfort of your own home.

Day 293 tip – Good food

Don't let a visit to the movie theatre become a horror show

The foods usually available when you're visiting a movie theatre can be a horror scene in themselves. A large bucket of popcorn supplies 35 grams of fat, which is more than you need in a whole day (and it's only a snack).

Not to mention the swimming pool sized portions of soft drink and the full-fat ice-cream choc top – you'd have to run for two hours instead of sitting still and watching the show just to burn it off.

Living it

Choose the bottled water or eat something healthy before you go to avoid temptation. If you must have junk, share it, go for small portions, and look for a small amount of the sugar-based sweets (musk sticks, snakes and jelly beans) instead of chocolate. You're probably not meant to smuggle your own healthy snacks into the cinema, but for the sake of your wellbeing it's a pretty good idea. You could take along some pretzels, air popped popcorn or rice crackers, and save yourself a whole lot of kilojoules. You can still enjoy the show without a full-scale assault on your healthy eating plan.

Day 294 tip – Move more

Give your walking some stick

Using your arms to propel you forwards with two ski poles while you walk is also known as Nordic walking, and it's one of the latest exercise fads. The poles make walking more of a whole body workout, using more upper body and abdominal muscles than regular walking. Developed by cross-country skiers to build their endurance and strength in the off-season, Nordic walking helps you to walk faster and burn more fat without hardly even noticing the extra effort. Nordic walking has been shown to increase the amount of kilojoules you burn by up to 45% when compared to regular walking. It also helps to increase your heart rate by around 5–15 beats more per minute.

Living it

If you're looking to add a whole new dimension to your exercise routine, and reduce the impact placed on your lower body, this could be for you. If you're worried about looking a little silly, share in the fun with a friend or get out in the bush where you can find your own space. The poles can be used on asphalt, sand or grass.

Day 295 tip – Motivation and mindset

Don't attempt to lose weight and quit smoking at the same time

Research has shown that when smokers quit they gain an average of around 3.5 kilograms over the following 12 months. There are a number of reasons why quitting causes weight gain, suggesting it may not be a good idea to make these two lifestyle changes at the same time. For all its damaging effects on people's health, nicotine actually speeds up the metabolic rate, and this drops considerably after quitting. Smoking also suppresses the senses of taste and smell, so when people quit, food can smell and taste better. Women are more likely to crave fatty foods when they quit. People also substitute smoking with snacking, finding comfort in a new activity involving the hands and mouth. Even so, research has shown that you are healthier being a fat non-smoker than a thin smoker.

Living it

Smoking is a very hard habit to break, and it may be better to lose weight first. This is because you are more likely to feel positive about giving up smoking after making other improvements in your health, and you don't have to face two major lifestyle changes at the one time.

Day 296 tip – Good food

If you enjoy pizza, make it yourself

There's no doubting the popularity of pizza, but when just two slices of a commercial variety bring around 30 grams of fat, it's certainly not going to help you lose weight.

Living it

There are a number of ways you can make a pizza healthy without sacrificing too much taste, especially by cutting out the fatty meats and cheese. Use these guidelines when ordering a pizza, or even better, make it yourself.

Instead of ...	Go for ...
Thick base, cheese stuffed crust	Thin base, wholemeal pizza base
Coating the pizza tray heavily in oil	Thin coating of cooking spray, or no oil on the tray
Pepperoni, salami, sausage, bacon	Shredded chicken breast, lean lamb strips, ham, prawns
Extra cheese, full-fat cheese	Minimal or no cheese, or use a low-fat cheese
Large portions	Small portions plus a garden salad
Garlic bread	Garden salad (you get bread with the pizza)
Meat toppings	Vegetable toppings, such as capsicum, tomato, pink onion, roasted pumpkin, roasted eggplant, mushrooms

Day 297 tip – Move more

Include running in your exercise program (conditions apply)

Very few activities burn as many kilojoules as running. The extra intensity can add some real impact to your workouts, even if you don't run the whole way. Running is very effective at boosting your metabolic rate, so you can get a much better workout in less time compared to walking. If you're comfortable with the thought of running (many people can't even bear to think about it), maybe it's something you should try.

Living it

The pros and cons of running depend upon your weight and level of fitness. Include more jogging or running in your training program if you:

- can walk comfortably for an hour at a fast pace
- weigh less than 100 kilograms
- are reasonably fit
- don't have existing knee problems.

Start with short runs during your walks and build up from there. Wear shoes with good cushioning and run on sand or grass occasionally to lessen the impact on your joints.

Day 298 tip – Motivation and mindset

Cultivate your emotional intelligence

Emotional intelligence has nothing to do with how smart you are. It's about your ability to manage the emotions such as fear, envy, sadness and worry that steer our day-to-day lives. In regards to weight management, it's about understanding the reasons and emotions behind any overeating or inactivity. Most people are smart enough to understand the importance of nutrition and exercise, but spend very little time on self-awareness and self-management. If you're eating but not hungry, or inactive even though you want to lose weight, there are probably underlying reasons why you are self-sabotaging.

Living it

You have the time, the knowledge and the desire to lose weight, but you need to make a connection between your emotions and your behaviour. You can work on and develop the emotional tools to help manage your weight, including the following.

- **Become self-motivated** – Direct yourself towards a goal, despite any inertia or self-doubts.

- **Become self-aware** – Know how to control yourself and your emotions. Recognise emotions as they occur and look for healthy ways to deal with them.

- **Manage your moods** – Deal with the ups and downs, but realise they are temporary. Keep them relevant to the current situation and don't let them interfere with other parts of your life.

- **Manage relationships** – Resolve conflicts and develop your ability to communicate and co-operate with others.

Day 299 tip – Good food

Grow your own herbs and vegetables

Having your own fresh herbs and vegetables will really encourage you to eat more plant foods, which in turn will help reduce your kilojoule intake. Not only will your own herb and veggie garden save money, it will add a fresh, fat-free flavour to all your healthy recipes. Even if you live in a small apartment, you can still grow herbs in pots on the balcony or windowsill.

Living it

Start with herbs and vegetables that are easy to grow like parsley, mint, chives, shallots, rosemary, lettuce, spinach and bok choy. You'll soon have the unique satisfaction that comes with using your own home grown herbs and vegetables in your meals. What's more, you'll even burn a few extra kilojoules preparing, weeding and watering your garden.

Day 300 tip – Move more

Sign up for boot camp

Boot camp is a group-based, military style outdoor training program designed to help you lose fat and increase your cardiovascular fitness. Sessions are usually held in a park, or at a beach, and will challenge you both physically and mentally. There are usually two or three sessions each week for a set number of weeks, and they are held rain, hail or shine. Most programs will cater for different levels of fitness and will include a range of activities, such as running, intervals, hill training, stair climbing, push-ups, sit-ups, lunges, core strengthening, team challenges and fitness tests.

Living it

If you like the thought of a little extra discipline and intensity with your exercise, plus some fresh air and the support of like-minded people, boot camp could be for you. The trainers will watch your every move, and push you harder than you are likely to push yourself. Boot camp will also keep you accountable because a whole group of people will know when you don't show up for your workout. You could also get together a group of friends and form your own boot camp.

Day 301 tip – Motivation and mindset

Avoid things that de-motivate you

Just as I encourage you use to strategies that motivate you, I also encourage you to identify and avoid the things that de-motivate you. These are the sorts of things that make you exhausted or uninspired, leaving you drained and unable to put in the effort you normally can. Everyone has them, and they can quickly turn from a small speed hump into a massive barrier when they stack up.

Living it

Try to identify the things that de-motivate you, and do your best to prevent them. Here are some of the more common de-motivators:

- negative attitude
- continually focusing on your results
- expectations of fast results
- comparisons with others
- negative people
- keeping 'fat' clothes
- tiredness from lack of sleep
- injury
- busy schedule
- food binges.

Day 302 tip – Good food

You don't have to clean your plate (but eat your veggies)

Do you eat everything that's put in front of you? It's a lesson most of us were taught as kids and it's a hard one to let go of. The concept is outdated now because many portion sizes, especially those served at restaurants, are excessive. Research has shown that the more food served, the more people eat, even if it exceeds kilojoule needs. Another study showed that the amount of food served was more important in determining kilojoule intake than what was eaten previously, or the fat, protein or carbohydrate content of their food. Finishing what's on your plate has evolved to be more important than our own self-regulating signals from the stomach to the brain. This is especially evident when people eat out at restaurants, feeling they need to finish what's on their plate to get value. It seems that humans are good at eating when they are hungry but not very good at stopping when there're full.

Living it

Don't put more food on your plate than you need. Try to serve smaller portions, eat off a smaller plate, and learn to listen to your body when it comes to food. You can still enjoy your food and the company of others without eating until you're uncomfortable. Another solution is to fill out your meals by adding low-kilojoule foods like vegetables.

Day 303 tip – Move more

Train for an event or fun run

Organised walks, swims, cycle events and fun runs are a great way to inject some enthusiasm into your exercise program. These events are great for weight loss because they give you a goal to train for, and an excuse to push yourself a little harder than normal. These events are usually open to all ages and fitness levels, and typically include options for different course lengths and starting times.

Living it

Training for an organised event can be motivating and fun. Why not look into participating in an event in your local area. If you become a regular participant, you'll have a time to beat each year. There may also be an opportunity to go along with friends, workmates or your family. Don't be intimidated about exercising in a crowd or feel you have to jog in a fun run. You can walk, jog or run at your own pace.

Day 304 tip – Motivation and mindset

Part ways with your yo-yo

No, not the toy! Yo-yo dieting, or weight cycling, is defined as periods of standard eating followed by crash dieting and bingeing, causing frequent and dramatic changes in body weight. People can get caught in a cycle of dieting, weight loss, weight regain, weight increase, more desperate dieting and further attempts at weight loss. Research has shown that in addition to shortening your lifespan, yo-yo dieting slows down your metabolic rate, making it harder to lose weight again in the future. There have even been reports to indicate that crash dieting can induce an early menopause. But it's not just the physical consequences, it's also the discouragement and disappointment that comes with another failed attempt.

Living it

No diet is successful if the weight loss doesn't last. If you can't stick to a diet over the long-term and maintain your results, that diet has failed you. You haven't failed the diet. Avoid extreme diets; they might seem beneficial in the short–term but they only make things worse in the long-term. Don't start any new diet trick, pattern or program unless you can picture yourself doing it for more than a month. Focus a healthy eating plan with gradual changes and expect a gradual weight loss. That way you can avoid a gradual return to your old weight.

Day 305 tip – Good food

Eat more of this weight resistant fibre

Resistant starch is a type of carbohydrate that resists digestion in the small bowel and arrives undigested into the large bowel. Once there, it is 'fermented' by bacteria and results in the formation of fatty acids which are absorbed into the bloodstream; and they have some proven weight-loss benefits. A study showed that resistant starch can increase fat oxidation by 23%, changing the order in which the body burns food. Usually carbohydrates are used first, but when resistant starch is present, dietary fat is oxidised first into energy before it has a chance to be stored as body fat. Other benefits for weight control include a reduced need for insulin, improved sensitivity to insulin and increased fullness.

Living it

One of the best sources of resistant starch is called Hi-Maize, which comes from a special strain of corn. You can find it added to breads, pasta and breakfast cereals without altering the taste, colour or texture of the food. You can also buy it at health food shops and use it instead of flour. Other sources of resistant starch include:

- intact wholegrain cereals, seeds and nuts, such as oats, rye, wheat, barley, semolina, corn, linseed, sesame
- legumes such as lentils and baked beans are a very good source of resistant starch
- unripe fruit, especially bananas

- cooking and cooling carbohydrate foods can also increase their resistant starch content, such as cold rice (sushi), cold pasta salad and potato salad.

Day 306 tip – Move more

Try a team sport, or group activity

There are myriad activities out there for every level of fitness and sporting ability, including volleyball, basketball, soccer, touch football and tennis. You might even consider group classes of jazzercise, cycling, aerobics and walking. They all give you the opportunity to improve your fitness and strength and burn significant amounts of kilojoules. But they offer you much more in other areas, such as fun, teamwork, social interaction and learning new skills. You tend to develop a higher level of unwavering commitment towards group activities than you would do yourself, which is great for your motivation to persist and push yourself harder.

Living it

Get involved in group activities as much as you can and push yourself a little harder. These types of activities add real variety to your routine, and in some ways you won't even feel like you're exercising. But some activities like ball sports have a higher risk of injury due to the short burst of exertion and lateral movements, which place extra demands on your muscles, ligaments and joints. So warm up properly, strengthen the appropriate muscle for your chosen activity, and stretch afterwards.

Day 307 tip – Motivation and mindset

Take some time out at a health retreat

If you want to try something different and kick-start your results, you could always visit a health retreat. You can experience a wide range of exercise classes and activities, get advice from a range of health professionals, attend lectures and cooking classes on healthy eating, or unwind with a massage. Some retreats also address the emotional and psychological aspects of weight loss. Meals tend to be vegetable based, but most people genuinely enjoy the creative and tasty foods on offer. You may even come home with a new batch of recipes. Many of the retreats are located in picturesque settings, offering you a tranquil space to get away from the rigours of everyday life.

Living it

Before you stay at a health retreat, make sure to choose one that best fits your needs. Make sure the focus is on exercise and healthy eating to achieve weight loss. It should be a place where you feel comfortable, so you can focus on getting your health in order.

- -

Day 308 tip – Good food

Don't waste your time on a low-carbohydrate diet

There's no doubting the popularity of low-carbohydrate diets, and they do work (on the scales). But the weight people lose on low-carb diets like the Atkins Diet is often muscle as well as fat, and rarely does the weight loss last. Carbohydrates are stored with a lot of water in your muscles, so when you cut them out, your weight loss on the scales can be quite dramatic. However, as soon as you go off the diet (and you will because they make you feel ordinary), the water is reloaded into your muscles, and any weight you've lost will almost certainly come back. Fast weight loss means fast weight regain. Research has also shown that low-carbohydrate diets have a very low compliance rate. In other words, people can't stick with them.

Living it

Why start something you almost know you won't stick to. Carbohydrates are an essential source of fuel for an active body, and it's more important to watch your portions and focus on improving the quality of your carbohydrates (lowering their GI) instead of eliminating them. Cut back on your carbs, but don't cut them out.

- -

Day 309 tip – Move more

Dance yourself slim

Is dancing enough of an exercise to help with weight loss? It is, depending on how long, how vigorous and how often you do it. Dancing is an enjoyable, social activity that has the added benefit of being good for your health. One recent study found that square dancers covered up to 8 kilometres in a single evening of dancing. To burn fat, you need to accumulate at least 30 minutes of moderately intense physical activity on most, preferably all days of the week. Most dancing classes last more than 30 minutes, but it's unlikely people would dance on most days of the week. The other important factor, intensity, varies considerably between dancing styles. Intensive types of dancing will certainly elevate your heart rate and help burn fat, yet there are many other types of dancing where the music, and pace, is slower.

Living it

Dancing can burn lots of kilojoules and help you burn fat. To get started, choose a style of dancing that you enjoy or would like to try and find the nearest dance centre where you can learn. Start gradually and your dancing, self-confidence and fitness will grow as you begin to master a new skill. Combine it with other activities like fast walking or slow jogging as part of balanced exercise plan.

Day 310 tip – Motivation and mindset

If you snore, lose 10% more

We know that poor quality sleep leads to weight gain, but weight gain can also lead to poor quality sleep. One of the main causes of snoring is excess fat around the mouth, tongue and jowls, which reduces the space for air to flow and increases the vibration in the throat. Heavy snorers can also suffer from sleep apnoea, where the airway becomes partially or completely collapsed during sleep. These temporary stoppages in breathing result in low oxygen levels and fragmented sleep, and can occur hundreds of times a night. It's estimated that up to 10% of the population (mostly male) suffer from sleep apnoea, but most are unaware of it.

Living it

If you snore, losing body fat will improve your quality of sleep and quality of life. Research has shown that losing 10% of your body fat will reduce your snoring by 30%. Cutting back on alcohol could also prove beneficial, and not just to help you lose weight. Alcohol causes your airway muscles to relax, so try not to drink just before going to bed.

Day 311 tip – Good food

Enjoy low-fat yoghurt (conditions apply)

Different varieties of yoghurt can range from a healthy snack to having enough sugar and fat to be classified as a dessert. The labels are also very confusing, with most popular 'diet', 'lite' or 'low fat' yoghurts containing over seven teaspoons of sugar in each 200 gram serve, and more kilojoules than full-fat plain yoghurt. For example, one brand that promotes itself as '94% fat-free' has 1346 kilojoules per 200 gram tub, whereas normal full-fat plain yoghurt contains 608 kilojoules. Normal full-fat yoghurt contains 3.4 grams per 100 grams, so try to ignore the labels and percentage claims. On the other hand, low-fat natural yoghurt is a great snack alternative to chips, biscuits and chocolate. In one study, obese people on a low-kilojoule diet who included three 170 gram servings of low-fat yoghurt daily for 12 weeks lost 22% more weight than dieters who ate little or no dairy. Importantly, they also lost 60% more body fat and maintained more lean muscle mass.

Living it

Use the nutrition information panel when selecting low-fat natural yoghurt, and look for brands with less than 500 kilojoules per 200 gram serve. You can then add your own fresh fruit to get some fibre with your sweetness, and also benefit from the weight reducing benefits of calcium and protein in the yoghurt.

Day 312 tip – Move more

Paddle your way to a better body

A good exercise that gives your lower body a rest while still burning plenty of fat and kilojoules is paddling. It's a great way to train while enjoying the great outdoors and spending time on the water. It will strengthen and tone your upper body while also strengthening the core if you use your torso while paddling. Just 20 minutes burns off around 500 kilojoules.

Living it

Why not look into kayaking (single or double), rowing, canoeing or rafting? There are many places that hire out paddle craft, so you can enjoy some time on the water at minimal expense. Also growing in popularity is dragon boating, which emphasises team spirit and fun. It's easy to learn and can be very motivating when you have a crew of 20 to keep up with.

Day 313 tip – Motivation and mindset

Don't waste your money on cellulite creams and cures

Cellulite is a natural condition, mostly found in women, caused by fat deposits pushing up between tiny ligaments running from the skin's surface, giving that dimpled appearance on the thighs, butt and hips. Cellulite looks identical under a microscope to body fat from any other part of your body. A combination of factors may contribute to cellulite, such as sluggish circulation, ineffective tissue drainage, excess body fluids, a slow metabolism, loss of skin elasticity, and stress. This can enlarge skin cells and contribute to the lumps and bumps. No cream, rub or lotion has proven to be effective in the removal of cellulite. It is not possible to massage or exercise a specific area in order to move, break up, burn or detoxify that area. Cellulite can occur on skinny people and larger people, and you can't get rid of it; but a healthy lifestyle can make it appear less obvious.

Living it

The principles for the removal of cellulite are identical to the principles of fat loss outlined in this book. There is no special treatment, cream, massage, exercise or diet, although cutting back on salt and alcohol may further reduce fluid retention and improve the appearance of cellulite.

Day 314 tip – Good food

Shrink your stomach (naturally)

You've probably heard of surgical procedures such as stomach stapling, stomach bypass and lap banding which reduce the quantity of food that can enter the stomach, helping you lose weight. But significant weight loss doesn't have to mean drastic solutions. Let's go to the world of science. Research has shown that overeating and consuming large individual meals on a regular basis can stretch the stomach wall, increasing your capacity to eat more. Some obese people have 40% more stomach capacity than lean people. Additional research suggests that by cutting down on the amount of food you eat, it is possible to shrink your stomach so you feel full after eating less food. Overweight subjects put on a very low-kilojoule diet for 4 weeks lost an average of 9 kilograms and decreased their gastric capacity, or the amount of liquid their stomachs could hold, by an average of 27%.

Living it

Your stomach is a muscular organ that expands temporarily when you eat then returns to its normal size afterwards. How much our stomach can stretch or shrink permanently is probably open for more research, but there are some informed things you can do.

- Retrain your stomach by gradually eating less, helping your body get used to smaller portions.

- Put up with a little hunger for a week or two as your body gets used to smaller portions.

- Drink a glass of cold water before eating, which is thought to slightly shrink your stomach, making you less hungry.

- Eat slowly and chew your food thoroughly.

- Avoid binges and large feasts that stretch your stomach to its capacity.

Day 315 tip – Move more

Jump towards a better body with a trampoline

Jumping on a trampoline is a great way to burn fat and get fit, helping to burn kilojoules, work your muscles, increase your heart rate, and improve your balance. The new breed of circular trampolines are surrounded by a nylon mesh, making them significantly safer than the traditional rectangular trampolines with exposed springs. A cheaper and more mobile alternative is the mini-trampoline that you can bounce on while watching television.

Living it

Trampolines come in all shapes and sizes, and there are options for all budgets, ages and abilities. They are especially beneficial if you struggle with any impact through the joints in your lower body. The larger trampolines can be a good investment for your whole family, while the mini-trampolines are good choice if you are looking for a cheap, quiet and comfortable exercise option for those days you don't want to venture outside.

Day 316 tip – Motivation and mindset

Have genuine enthusiasm for your pursuit of better health

When it comes to losing weight and changing your lifestyle, results usually come in proportion to the enthusiasm that's applied. If knowledge is power, enthusiasm turns on the switch. A little extra enthusiasm can make all the difference between success and failure. Being enthusiastic means that you never let a day go by without doing something that moves you towards your goal. Maintaining that enthusiasm will prove to be a dynamic and motivating force that raises you above anything you have achieved before.

Living it

As the saying goes, the only difference between try and triumph is just a little 'umph'. The key to harnessing and developing enthusiasm is to incorporate the character traits of passionate people. Here are some ways you can develop a little more passion and enthusiasm about losing weight and body fat.

- **Forget about yesterday** – Leave mistakes in the past, and be enthusiastic about the now.
- **Believe in yourself** – Don't hold back because you don't think you have the ability, or the right, to achieve success. You are worthy and

capable, and possessing just as much potential as anyone else who has reached their goals.

- **Be inspired** – Spend time with and learn from the people who have already achieved the same goals as you. Their enthusiasm will rub off.

- **Focus single-mindedly on what you want** – Having clarity about what you want to achieve and how you're going to achieve it helps to generate determination, positive thinking and concentration. Setbacks become less significant when you stay focused on the big picture.

- **Make a commitment** – People who have a burning desire to succeed will do whatever it takes to get there, even if it means cutting back on a few indulgences.

Day 317 tip – Good food

Enjoy your pasta (conditions apply)

Pasta is a very popular food, and it can be a help or a hindrance to your weight-loss efforts depending on a few variables. Pasta is much more likely to be fattening if your portion sizes are high and your activity levels are low. Excess kilojoules from any type of food will be stored as fat, and pasta is no exception. Look for wholemeal pasta, which contains more nutrients and has a low GI to keep you feeling sustained for longer. The other thing to watch out for is the company pasta keeps.

Living it

Follow these guidelines so you can enjoy pasta without it being a kilojoule disaster.

Instead of ...	Go for ...
White pasta	Wholemeal pasta
Meat and pasta sauces	Meat and pasta sauces with lots of added vegetables
Creamy pasta sauces	Tomato pasta sauces
Oil in the sauce or in the pasta to stop it clinging	Minimal oil, and rapidly boiling water to stop pasta clinging
Garlic bread	Wholegrain bread roll
Large portions	Smaller portions of pasta, and include a garden salad
Topping with yellow cheese	Topping with a minimal amount of strong cheese such as parmesan
Alcohol	Water, a small glass of wine

Day 318 tip – Move more

Box your way to a better body

Cardioboxing has grown in stature over recent years to become one of the most popular forms of exercise. It gives you a great upper body workout, not to mention the energy boost and stress relief from hitting something. Incorporating kickboxing moves and leg movements such as squats, jumps and kicks with boxing will use more muscles, and give you an even better fat-burning workout. A good boxing workout can burn over 2000 kilojoules in just 45 minutes, which is much higher than most other activities.

Living it

You can do boxing and kickboxing at many different levels, from a few basic pieces of equipment at home, to DVDs and fitness classes, to sparring and full-contact sport. Some of the DVDs and classes combine elements of boxing, kickboxing, martial arts and aerobics for total conditioning and fat burning, and can be a good starting point. It's really a matter of choosing a style that suits you. Whatever you choose, boxing has significant weight-loss benefits, especially if you incorporate leg movements.

Day 319 tip – Motivation and mindset

Learn to spot a scam

For every complicated problem such as weight loss there is often a simple solution – and rarely does that simple solution work. There is no simple, quick fix for weight loss. But that doesn't stop people offering simple solutions, and trying to make money. Just recently, a new diet book touted the benefits of eating butter, cream and raw (unpasteurised) milk, based on the diets of isolated tribes in the 1920s (and the relevance of this to modern life still escapes me). These diet claims attract media attention because they go against traditional advice. But that doesn't make them right.

Living it

If you answer yes to any of these questions, you can be pretty sure you've found another slimming scam.

- Does it claim that you don't have to exercise?
- Are there recommendations to sell a product or supplement?
- Are there warnings such as 'results not typical' or 'must be combined with exercise and a kilojoule-controlled diet'?
- Does it encourage you to cut out whole food groups or include items you can't normally buy at the supermarket?

- Are you encouraged to do something at a certain time, such as only eat fruit till midday, or no grapefruit on Wednesdays?
- Do the claims sound too good to be true?
- Is the program or advice questioned by well-known scientific organisations or experts?
- Is it a program that you would find hard to stick to over the long-term?

Day 320 tip – Good food

Follow this handy tip for portion size

Keeping your portion size down is one of the 10 commandments for fat loss, but it can be hard to measure. Many people underestimate the amount of food they eat and overestimate the recommended portion sizes for many foods. That's why it helps to relate your serving sizes to everyday items, to help visualise what a true portion size looks like.

Living it

Considering your hand should be with you everywhere you go, here are some helpful comparisons.

- Make a fist and look at the size of it because it's a good indicator of the capacity of your stomach, no matter what frame size you are. This is the amount of food (after chewing) that you need to feel satisfied, but it's not enough to feel stuffed. Use it as a guide for your entire meal.
- The palm of your hand (don't count your fingers) is a good guide for a serving of meat such as a small chicken breast, lean beef or fish fillet.
- The tip of your thumb is a useful guide to a teaspoon of oil or a teaspoon of peanut butter.
- The whole of your thumb (tip to base) is a good guide for a serving of hard yellow cheese or a snack of some nuts.

Day 321 tip – Move more

Take a hike with your exercise routine

Bushwalking gives you the chance to tackle a variety of outdoor tracks and cross-country paths while taking in the best that nature has to offer. It's also a great way to escape from modern life and get some air in your lungs. It costs next to nothing and you can choose the terrain to suit your level of fitness – from gentle undulating hills and trails to rugged mountain peaks. Long walks should burn a significant amount of fat and the uneven terrain is a good change from the road, park or treadmill. It's been estimated that you can burn 33% more kilojoules bushwalking than by walking on level surfaces.

Living it

Whether you go hiking through our national parks or just trek through some local bushland, it's a great way to get close with nature, spend time with friends and family, and burn off some kilojoules. Make sure you wear good-quality footwear with enough tread to make you feel steady on your feet. Also pack plenty of water and healthy snacks. Why not get out and explore this weekend.

Day 322 tip – Motivation and mindset

Manage your anger to manage your weight

Do you find yourself shouting at your kids more than you'd like or responding aggressively to situations when you shouldn't? You're not alone; research shows there is a growing trend in social incidents such as road rage, surf rage and trolley rage. The research also shows that this could be having a negative effect on your body shape. People who lose their temper are more likely to be overweight, which relates to another study that showed overweight people were 50% more likely to use food to cope with emotions such as anger.

Living it

It's important to note that dysfunctional anger is not to blame for the current obesity epidemic, but it can be one piece of the weight-loss puzzle that needs to be addressed. You may not be able to change the situations and events that frustrate you, but you can change how you react to them. Anger is a strong emotion, but you can learn to manage it and even harness it for your benefit. Consider purchasing a punching bag and gloves to release some frustrations, or go for a walk to cool down. Or try relaxation techniques, improving your communication skills, using humour, changing your environment or seeking counselling.

Day 323 tip – Good food

Drink green tea to accelerate fat burning

Green tea is the least processed type of tea, which preserves an antioxidant known as epigallocatechin gallate (EGCG). There are a number of proven benefits from drinking green tea, but let's look at its weight-loss and fat-burning properties. EGCG (not found in black tea) speeds up your brain and nervous system, just like caffeine revs up your heart rate. Research has shown that green tea can boost your metabolic rate more than caffeine, and increase the number of daily kilojoules you burn. A study compared daily kilojoule use after having three servings of caffeine, green tea or a dummy supplement. The green tea drinkers burned 1000 kilojoules more than the placebo group (an increase of 35%) and used a much higher proportion of fat as fuel than both other groups.

	Daily kilojoules	Fat kilojoules
Placebo	9572	2881
Caffeine	9631	3095
Green tea	9899	3893

Living it

Not only does green tea accelerate weight loss, it tastes good. You can also add a little lemon to improve its taste without affecting the antioxidant (EGCG) levels. A little green tea before exercise can help you burn more kilojoules, and is well worth a try.

Day 324 tip – Move more

Get on your bike, and burn off fat

Cycling is a great outdoor addition to your exercise program for burning fat and aerobic conditioning. While not as effective as running or walking for fat loss because your weight is supported by the seat, you can still burn off a significant amount of kilojoules if you aim for longer sessions of exercise. Bikes also allow you to take in much more scenery in the time that you invest in exercise, so it can be a great mind–body experience.

Living it

To emphasise weight and fat loss, use an easy gear or low level of resistance and aim for a fast pedalling speed. Harder levels of resistance, hills and intervals can also add variety and intensity to your cycling. An on-board computer is a good addition, allowing you to monitor your speed, average speed, distance covered, duration and kilojoules used. Just make sure you don't skimp on safety gear, like an approved helmet, reflectors and a light if you ride at night. Another option is an indoor trainer, which supports the bike on rollers and instantly converts your outdoor bike into an indoor exercise bike.

Day 325 tip – Motivation and mindset

Forget about what French women do. Nearly half of them are fat

Contrary to what you may have read or heard, French women do get fat. A study has shown that at least 40% of French citizens are overweight or obese, which is not so far behind Australia. It's also not surprising from a country famous for its pastries, cheese and champagne. If you eat more kilojoules than you burn off, you'll gain weight – no matter where you live. The French are not immune from weight problems, with skyrocketing rates of childhood obesity, just like many other industrialised nations.

Living it

While it's important to make fat loss all about you and ignore what the Joneses are doing, French women do have lower levels of body fat, and set some good examples with their eating. Firstly, huge portion sizes, fast food and overly processed products are the exception rather than the norm. The lesson to eat foods for pleasure, and truly savour small portions is a good one. Eat moderate portions slowly, eat plenty of healthy nourishing foods and don't deprive yourself of what you enjoy. Merci.

Day 326 tip – Good food

Don't worry about going gluten free (conditions apply)

Gluten is a protein found in wheat, rye, and other cereals, and it has become the subject of diet books and much debate in recent times. Gluten can cause a range of unpleasant digestive problems in people who are either gluten intolerant, or who suffer varying degrees of coeliac disease. This has resulted in the wide range of gluten-free products now available on supermarket shelves. While people with coeliac disease must follow a gluten-free diet, other people who haven't even been diagnosed with the disease are going gluten-free, believing it will help them lose weight.

Living it

Because gluten is found in wheat, barley, rye and oats, the list of foods you have to avoid is extensive. Cutting back on grain-based foods will help reduce your kilojoule intake and lose weight, but you don't need to cut them out if your body can tolerate gluten. Some gluten-free products are actually high in sugar, or have a higher GI because they are made from rice or potato flour, so they are not necessarily a better choice for weight loss. If you suspect you have some of the symptoms of coeliac disease, such as fatigue, diarrhoea, flatulence and bloating, discuss it with your doctor, who can give you a test for the disease.

Day 327 tip – Move more

Give rollerblading a try

There's plenty to like about rollerblading (sometimes called inline skating). Like all exercises, the faster and harder you go, the more kilojoules you'll burn. Studies have shown that rollerblading is on par with running as a kilojoule-burning activity, with half the impact and triple the fun. It was also rated as a better cardiovascular workout than cycling because even when you coast along, you are still standing up. It also tones and strengthens the entire upper leg, buttocks and abdominals, while the muscles in your upper arms and shoulders will get a workout depending on how vigorously you swing your arms. It's also one of the few exercises that targets your inner and outer thighs.

Living it

Rollerblading can be done on a quiet road, bike path, footpath or any smooth, safe place to skate on. The best place to start is probably with a lesson, where you can hire some rollerblades and safety gear and try before you buy. You'll also pick up a few handy tips that will get you on your way. This is a fairly challenging activity at first, but once you get the knack of it, you've found an excellent weekend kilojoule burner. Avoid any uphill or downhill sections until your skills develop.

Day 328 tip – Motivation and mindset

Face facts on surgical solutions

For cases of severe obesity, there is an argument for surgical procedures such as stomach lap banding as a last-ditch solution. A small belt is surgically inserted around the stomach, which can then be adjusted using a fine needle to inject or withdraw fluid. There may be three or four adjustments in the first year after the procedure to further barricade the stomach and reduce its food capacity, or relax it to ease restrictions, depending on the patient's results. It's a desperate remedy, with a death rate between one or two per thousand, but the consequences of inaction may be even more desperate.

Living it

A major concern is the advertising of this procedure by some clinics as a weight-loss solution for anyone.

It's best reserved for people who are extremely overweight, and who are suffering serious health conditions such as diabetes or sleep apnoea.

Patients have to be very co-operative and follow a liquid diet for a week or two, after which purees and solids can be reintroduced. Food intake has to be in small portions because overeating will cause vomiting, while some foods such as bread and red meat may never be properly tolerated. It usually results in steady, and relatively slow weight loss over 2 or 3 years.

Day 329 tip – Good food

Go for the good oil (but not too much)

Olive oil is extremely high in kilojoules (just like all other fats and oils), but small portions can add interest and flavour to a healthy, weight reducing diet. While it's important to keep your fat intake down, olive oil is one of the best choices to make when you do have fat. Olive oil helps to slow down the absorption of carbohydrates, reducing your body's need to release insulin. Olive oil is also beneficial for your heart, and it's thought to be partly responsible for the low levels of heart disease in people from Mediterranean countries. The benefits come from its high mono-unsaturated fat content, and because extra virgin olive oil is minimally processed, it retains the fruit's natural antioxidants and other nutrients. Just like wine, the flavour of olive oil can vary dramatically depending on the type of olive, climate, soil and the blend. Olive oil comes in different varieties, depending on how much it's processed, and includes:

- **Extra virgin** – The first, cold or unheated press of the fruit, which retains the most taste, aroma, vitamins and nutrients of the olive.

- **Pure** – After the first pressing, more oil is extracted using some heating and processing.

- **Light/extra light** – This is not lower in kilojoules but is highly processed using a combination of pressure, heat, filtering and chemicals. This removes most of the colour, odour and taste, making it more suitable for frying and baking.

Living it

When you do eat fats, watch your portions, and look for those with the least amount of processing, such as extra virgin olive oil. You could say that it's one of the least fattening fats. Enjoy it as Mediterranean people do, at room temperature over breads, salads and vegetables. This prevents the formation of dangerous trans fatty acids, which occur when oils are heated during cooking.

Day 330 tip – Move more

Join a gym, and actually go

Joining a gym has many advantages, as long as you feel comfortable in that environment, and you make the most of your membership. Having a gym membership supports your healthy lifestyle by giving you an option on cold, wet or windy days, and provides access to an incredible variety of exercises and equipment. You can try out some of the different types of floor classes, get into resistance training or use the cardiovascular machines. Some gyms are for women only or include special rooms just for women or personal training customers. Be aware that a lot of people are gym members but very rarely attend.

Living it

Before you join a gym, why not try before you buy. Ask for a free visit or pay $15–$20 for a one-off casual visit to get a feel for the place. You can then also be in a better position to rate the gym in these important criteria.

- Do you feel comfortable with the facility and other members?
- Do you feel comfortable with the staff? They should be friendly and helpful, not pushing you to join.
- Is the gym a well-established business?
- Is the location easy for you to use?
- Do they have a good selection of equipment that you want to use?
- Is the gym packed out at the main times you want to attend?
- Is the equipment clean and well maintained?
- Does the gym have lockers for your valuables?
- Are there childcare facilities?
- Is there plenty of parking?
- Can you put your membership on hold?
- Is the air fresh and well ventilated?
- How hot does it get in summer?

Day 331 tip – Motivation and mindset

Learn from the Japanese – the land of the lean

You won't see a lot of overweight people in Japan. In fact, they have some of the lowest overweight and obesity rates in the industrialised world.

Living it

Anyone can copy the dietary habits of Japanese people. See if you can make these habits your own.

- Base your diet on low-fat foods like fish, soya, rice, vegetables and fruit.
- Eat smaller portions, served in small bowls. The smaller your bowl, the less you will eat.
- Cook with less oil, and use healthy cooking methods like steaming, sautéing or simmering.
- Eat small amounts of rice (Basmati) with your meals instead of bread.
- Avoid flour-based products like muffins, pastries and white bread.
- Make breakfast your biggest, most protein-packed meal of the day to maximise your energy levels through to lunch.
- Enjoy the occasional dessert and treat, but keep your portions tiny.

Day 332 tip – Good food

Eat like you live in the Mediterranean

This style of eating originates from countries bordering the Mediterranean Sea, such as Spain, Greece and Italy. The emphasis is on good fats, good carbohydrates and taste. People who follow this style of eating have lower rates of heart disease and cancer, and there is growing evidence of its weight-loss benefits. People who will benefit most are those who currently have a diet high in saturated animal fats, and then switch to a Mediterranean diet high in mono-unsaturated fats. One study showed subjects who followed a Mediterranean diet lost more weight than those on a strictly low-fat diet. The good fats keep blood sugar levels balanced, and the high level of vitamins, minerals and antioxidants help the metabolism to function at its best.

Living it

There are plenty of reasons to eat Mediterranean. The following table gives you a better understanding of the typical foods consumed as part of a Mediterranean diet.

Eat mostly (nearly every day)	Vegetables, salads, beans and legumes, fruit, bread without butter or margarine, polenta and pasta, olive oil, red wine, nuts, seafood
Eat occasionally (a few times a week)	Eggs, poultry, fish, cheese, sweet foods
Eat rarely (monthly or less)	Butter, cream, red meat, processed meats

To achieve weight loss, modify the diet slightly by carefully watching your portion sizes for higher kilojoule foods such as oils, breads, pasta, cheese and alcohol. Try to only drink wine on the days you are active.

Day 333 tip – Move more

Take extreme measures and add variety to your exercise routine

If you want to take your exercise variety to the edge, you could always try some adventure activities. They burn kilojoules by paddling, peddling, climbing, jumping or just holding yourself in position. But it's not just about the kilojoules because these activities are about adrenaline, fun, excitement and pushing yourself to your limits. They can help you step out from your comfort zone, overcome your fears, and give you confidence that flows into other areas of your life. Some examples include:

- canyoning
- abseiling
- rock climbing
- climbing gyms
- mountain biking
- kite surfing
- bungee jumping
- snowboarding
- whitewater rafting.

Living it

These are the types of activities that won't necessarily be part of your regular cardiovascular training, but they are activities you can thrive at when exercise is a regular part of your life. You can try them at any age, but it will help to get some professional guidance when starting out to maximise your safety and enjoyment.

Day 334 tip – Motivation and mindset

Have more sex

A little roll in the hay can actually be pretty good exercise. You may have noticed that your heart beats faster, you puff and pant, you sweat and even feel a little exhausted afterwards, although the amount of physical effort expended during sex would vary dramatically. Research has shown (fun research) that pulse rate can be elevated as high as 170 heartbeats per minute during sex. It's also been estimated that a single act of intercourse may require as much physical effort as about 15 to 20 push-ups, and burn up to 1800 kilojoules per hour.

Living it

Even if you are lucky enough to get plenty of this type of physical activity, you can't rely on it alone to change your body shape. For some, there may be more kilojoules used in the chase than the doing. On the other hand, improving your cardiovascular fitness and muscle strength may actually improve your sexual performance by improving circulation for men and improving mood and libido in women. Either way, it's a type of exercise that won't require too much motivation.

Day 335 tip – Good food

Develop a bank of healthy recipes that you love

People have different tastes and reasons for eating, and there needs to be flexibility if you are going to stick with a healthy eating plan. There's no perfect diet, portion size, single meal (or soup) for everyone. Even so, there are some foods you should eat more of, and some you should eat less of if you want to lose weight.

Living it

Examine the breakfasts, lunches, dinners and snacks you eat over the course of an average fortnight, and you'll probably see the same meals and recipes cropping up time and time again. Dinners tend to vary the most, but even there you'll tend to have a few consistent favourites. There's nothing wrong with that, but for long-lasting weight loss it's important that these foundation recipes are healthy, low in kilojoules, and low in fat. Following the principles of healthy eating outlined in this book, experiment with new foods and recipe ideas, and gradually build up your repertoire of healthy meals and snacks. My hope is that you will discover a new collection of recipes and easy meals that taste great, and can form the foundation for lifelong healthy eating.

Day 336 tip – Move more

Dust off your skipping rope

Skipping is a great way to incorporate some high intensity activity into your day. You can have fun, get fit, burn fat, prevent osteoporosis and reduce your risk of heart disease all at the same time. Skipping has grown in popularity with the emergence of boxing training as a genuine path to fitness and fat loss. It's a convenient and cheap activity you can do anywhere, with the flexibility to make it harder or easier depending on your fitness level. Skipping is a high-impact activity, so it may not be suitable for people who have joint problems.

Living it

Start off slowly and aim for longer sessions of skipping with little jumps, which helps to minimise the impact on your knees and ankles. Skipping is fairly strenuous, so you may need frequent rests, when you can stretch or march on the spot while you catch your breath. As your fitness improves you can increase the amount of time you skip for, and reduce your rest periods. Go for a short walk afterwards to cool down and make sure to stretch your calf muscles.

Day 337 tip – Motivation and mindset

Don't look to celebrities for guidance

Sadly, our fascination with the rich and famous extends to their personal battles with diet, weight and body image. But you can't believe everything you see, and in some cases you wouldn't want to. Take Sylvester Stallone for example. He was in tremendous shape for Rocky 6, but the secret to his success was discovered by Australian customs officials (and anybody who was unfortunate enough to be walking by his hotel when vials of synthetic growth hormone were thrown out the window). I also know of a celebrity who gained a considerable amount of weight then auctioned themselves off to the highest bidding weight-control program as a weight-loss role model. Other celebrities can afford to have a full-time chef and exercise with a personal trainer 5 days a week, while some celebrity diets are bordering on dangerous.

Living it

While some celebrities look fantastic, you don't know to what extent airbrushing, surgical procedures, extreme training or dangerous dieting strategies are involved. By all means, use their success as motivation, but don't look to actors or singers for dietary advice. Look for more proven weight-loss guidance, with practical advice on nutrition, exercise, motivation and attitude from people qualified to give it.

Day 338 tip – Good food

Enjoy some different and unusual fruits

You'll probably find over 30 different types of fruits at your local supermarket, but how often does your shopping trolley see anything beyond the traditional apples, bananas and oranges? There are an increasing number of tasty, unusual fruits that are available all year round.

Living it

Fruit is a great snack, but don't get bored with the same old thing. You'll be less likely to revert back to junk food snacks like biscuits, chocolate or crisps if you can keep your healthy snacks interesting. Why not experiment with some varieties of fruits you haven't had for a while or never had before, such as these listed below.

- fresh figs
- loquats
- star fruits
- tangerines
- honeydew melon
- kumquats
- persimmon

- pomegranate
- guavas
- custard apples
- paw paw (papaya)
- mulberries
- lychees

Day 339 tip – Move more

Train for a triathlon

Why not throw yourself in the deep end – literally. There are few greater challenges in the world of exercise than competing in a triathlon. It's not just about getting fit for swimming, cycling and running, but you need to make time to train for three different activities. This may not appeal to everyone, but if you like to push yourself, it could open up a whole new world.

Living it

Find out the date of a triathlon within the next 12 months and mark it in your diary. Find out the distances for each leg of the triathlon and make a commitment to yourself. Start off very slowly, and build up your distances and times gradually. You can even create your own private triathlon with three activities of your choice or three cardiovascular machines at the gym.

Day 340 tip – Motivation and mindset

Don't worry about cleaning your liver. It can take care of itself

Let your liver take care of itself. Have you seen the liver tonics, supplements and special diets that promise to improve your liver function and melt away fat? It may seem like a simple solution, but in most cases, a faulty liver will not be the cause of weight gain or slow weight loss. We know that the liver can build up with fat in people who are diabetic or grossly overweight or drink large amounts of alcohol. But there is little evidence to support the claims that excess body fat is caused by a malfunctioning or unclean liver.

Living it

The liver is a self-cleaning organ and requires no special diet or herbal supplement to improve its effectiveness. A diet that includes nuts, seeds, avocado, soy foods, fish, fruit, vegetables and whole grains, and that eliminates alcohol, caffeine and animal fats will make you feel better. It doesn't have to be under the disguise of a special liver diet. Eating healthier, less processed foods will help your body function at its best (including your liver) and will also help you lose weight.

Day 341 tip – Good food

Rely on the occasional 'lean cuisine' or 'healthy choice'

While it's better to have prepared something yourself, there will be times when you are busy and tired and don't feel like cooking. These are the times when the convenience of fast food becomes tempting. But having a reasonably tasty and healthy meal in the freezer that can be ready in minutes could help to halve your kilojoule and fat intake (compared to choosing fast food). Just make sure you check the nutrition information panels because some frozen dinners are incredibly high in salt, kilojoules and fat.

Living it

While I won't rave about the benefits of frozen microwave dinners, 'lean cuisine' or 'healthy choice' offer some far better alternatives to hamburgers, pizza and fried chook. Don't live off them, but use them when you need a fast, cheap, portion- and kilojoule-controlled dinner. You can even add a few extra steamed vegetables.

Day 342 tip – Move more

Use a heart rate monitor to maximise fat burning

Heart rate monitors can be a great addition to your exercise routine. They allow you to continuously check your exercise intensity (heart rate), and make sure you are reaching the goal of a particular workout. They eliminate the guesswork out of measuring your training intensity, allowing you to increase or decrease your training level to maximise your chances of burning kilojoules and fat. Many models allow you to set training zones, which make a beeping sound if your heart rate strays from the desired performance level.

Living it

Calculate your maximum heart rate by subtracting your age from 220. If you are a beginner, keep your heart rate at 45–65% of your maximum. After a few weeks, go to 65–75% of your maximum. After a few months, work out at 75–85%, when you could also introduce intervals, where your heart rate may reach 85–95% of your maximum.

Day 343 tip – Motivation and mindset

Be a role model, and inspire others

It's often said that the best way to learn is to teach. As you work towards improving your lifestyle habits, try to encourage those around you to join in. Not only will you be helping the people close to you, but it will serve as extra motivation, knowing that there are people who look up to you and see you as a source of inspiration. You don't even have to say very much. Set an example, and people will see and learn that you can succeed at becoming healthier.

Living it

Try to be a healthy role model to your kids, friends, co-workers and family. Become a shining example of a lifestyle that radiates wellness. Eat well when it's easier not to, and exercise when all around you are asking how you find the time. When your actions inspire others to do more, learn more and become more, you share in their positive experiences.

Day 344 tip – Good food
Walk past the juice bar

Okay, so packaged fruit juice is not a good choice (see day 212). But what about juice bars, vegetable juices and freshly squeezed juice? I get asked this a lot, and often by the same people because they didn't like my answer the first time. The answer is simple – empty kilojoules. Squeezing, juicing or processing fruits and vegetables virtually eliminates the fibre and fullness potential of that food, no matter how fresh they are. All you are left with is little more than sugar and water, and a few more vitamins than you would find in a glass of cola. These liquid kilojoule explosions that are disguised as health drinks can really make it hard to get results. There is very little hunger satisfaction from all those kilojoules, which you still have to burn off before you'll burn off stored body fat.

Living it

You often see a juice bar positioned just outside a gymnasium, which is great if you are training to get fit or increase your weight. But in terms of fat loss, juice bar drinks are no different to having a soft drink. Have water, and eat your fruits and vegetables instead. If you must indulge, vegetable juices are a slightly better choice because they don't contain the sweetness (except for beetroot), so their kilojoule content is lower.

Day 345 tip – Move more
Periodise your training

Are you ready to take your cardiovascular exercise to a higher level? Once you have built a solid base of fitness, there's no reason why you can't use more advanced training technique to burn fat. Periodisation is a training method where you structure a program into distinct, separate phases to help you progress towards peak performance at a distant point in time. Various rates of volume and intensity are used to achieve results, although time is scheduled for physical and mental recovery.

Living it

Identify an event or set yourself a challenge to complete within the next 3–12 months. Some examples would be to compete in a fun run, triathlon or distance challenge that you set yourself. Between now and the date of completion, plan these five major phases to your training schedule.

- **The base** – Accumulate training time without too much intensity. Aim for 5–7 days a week and clock up a solid foundation of training

over a few months. It's a bit like a pyramid, the bigger the base the
higher the peak.

- **The build** – Begin training at a higher intensity on at least 3 days
  each week for 8–16 weeks. Include a fortnightly session where you
  push yourself over a similar time or distance that you will for your
  final event.

- **The taper** – Scale back your training in the week leading up to your
  event. You can still do a few light training sessions, but the idea is to
  face your event or challenge refreshed.

- **The race** – Time to actually compete in your event or challenge.
  You should be ready to give it your all.

- **The recovery** – Have some down time and take a week off from
  training. You can even use your time off to plan the training for your
  next challenge.

Day 346 tip – Motivation and mindset

Equip your kitchen with tools to support you

Your kitchen is an environment within your control, so it's important to
surround yourself with equipment that makes healthy cooking easier.

Living it

Get rid of the deep fryer and make room for these helpful items.

- **Non-stick pans and utensils** – Help to minimise the need for oil or
  fat and keep to your fat budget. Health grills, baking trays, fry pans,
  woks, muffin trays, pizza trays and cake tins are available with non-
  stick surfaces.

- **Food processors** – Save time and create different tastes and
  textures from food. Suitable for cutting up large amounts of
  vegetables, making sauces, dips and soups.

- **Blenders and mix masters** – Ideal for a quick snack in a glass.
  Fruit purees and smoothies are tasty and nutritious low-fat foods.

- **Non-stick baking paper** – This is a great product to help you
  minimise fat. The surface can be used as an alternative to butter,
  margarine or oil in a range of cooking applications, or you can
  parcel up and bake a whole meal, helping you cut back on
  kilojoules.

- **Good quality storage containers** – Have a variety of different sizes
  so you can keep your food fresh and freeze any leftovers and reheat
  them quickly in the microwave.

- **A good set of knives** – Make your cooking easier with a decent set of knives. Keep a sharpening tool close by so you can always slice your way through vegetables, lean meats and fresh herbs.

- **A steamer** – Steaming is one of the healthiest cooking techniques. There are different types of steamers for your pots or for the microwave.

- **Others** – Some other helpful items include an indoor grill, a salad spinner, a marinating brush, a grater, a citrus zester, a well-stocked spice rack and an organised recipe file.

Day 347 tip – Good food

Eat more berries – red, black and blue

Berries are top of the tree when it comes to health giving foods, including strawberries, raspberries, blackberries, cranberries and blueberries. The pigments that give berries their deep red, blue, black and purple colours make them one of the richest sources of antioxidants, which can help prevent heart disease and cancer. From a weight-loss perspective,

they are a good source of fibre and they are strongly flavoured, so you can get the taste without too many kilojoules.

Living it

There are so many varieties of berries, so it shouldn't be hard to find one you like. Their bright colours make them look appetising, and they taste great. Berries can be expensive, but you can always go for the frozen varieties so they last a while. Try them on your cereal, with yoghurt, in smoothies, as a snack, or as a dessert. As with all fruits, the whole package is always better than the juice.

Day 348 tip – Move more

Don't rely on swimming alone to help you lose weight

You are actually better off walking around a pool than swimming in it if you want to lose weight. Here's why:

- Your weight is supported by the water so fewer kilojoules are needed to help you move

- Fat floats, so the fatter you are the more you float and the fewer kilojoules you will use in water

- Women naturally have a higher proportion of fat to muscle and a lower centre of gravity than men; women actually float better in water, so they use fewer kilojoules than men

- Maintaining normal body temperature is much easier during and after swimming than during land-based activities; this reduces the increase in your metabolic rate and reduces the appetite suppressing effects of exercise.

Living it

Swimming is a good exercise for fitness and muscle tone, but there are better choices for weight and fat loss. On the other hand, it's far better than sitting on a couch and it's ideal for people with injuries or excessive weight who can't walk without pain.

Day 349 tip – Motivation and mindset

Once you've lost weight, keep it off

Would you believe me if I said that losing weight is the easy part? Have you lost weight and regained it in the past? Many people do, and research can back this up. One study showed that the kilograms you regain after losing a lot of weight can be particularly hard to shed again. A major issue with weight and fat loss maintenance is the changes in your kilojoule needs. Because there is physically less of you, your body needs less fuel, so when people resume their old diet after losing weight, it all comes back quite quickly. Physical activity is also vital. Your body uses fewer kilojoules during exercise when you weigh less, so it's important to continue to increase some or all of the parameters of exercise, such as the duration, frequency and intensity.

Living it

If you have reached a point where you are happy with your current level of body fat, don't surrender your healthy lifestyle and go back to how you were. Keep up your exercise program and healthy eating plan, and pay attention to small regains so they don't grow into large ones. Look for support groups, newsletters or magazines that help keep you informed and motivated.

Day 350 tip – Good food

Use a little peanut butter (conditions apply)

For peanut butter lovers, there's good news and bad news. The good news is that peanut butter is full of essential nutrients, protein and antioxidants. The bad news is that it's full of fat and kilojoules, with 1 tablespoon containing 400 kilojoules and 8 grams of fat. The other bad news is that the nutritious peanut butter probably won't be found in your supermarket aisles. Commercial peanut butters use processed oils to stop the oil from separating. Additional oils, salt and sugar may be also be added.

Living it

Peanut butter is high in fat and kilojoules and if fat loss is your goal, you don't want to eat it by the jarful. But it's also high in protein and fibre and has a low GI (especially the health food store varieties), so it will make you feel fuller for longer than a sugar-based spread such as jam or honey. If you want to include peanut butter in your diet, have it in small amounts, have it on multigrain bread and have it without butter or margarine. It's also great with a banana on toast or as a flavour additive to a vegetable stir-fry.

Day 351 tip – Move more

Take an active vacation

Just about any holiday can be turned into active travel, even if you spare an hour or two each day to lie about and do nothing. You should have more time than ever to keep to your exercise routine, and even try a whole new range of activities.

Living it

Make the most of your time away; consider some of these ideas on how to be more active on your next holiday.

- Pack your exercise shoes and use your feet. You can walk or run for some planned exercise, and walk instead of drive as you discover your new holiday destination.

- Why not challenge yourself and plan an active holiday where trekking, backpacking or sporting activities are an integral part of your getaway.

- Visit the local gym or fitness centre for a casual workout, or book into a hotel that has its own exercise equipment.

- Focus your entertainment and time with friends and family around non-food related activities, such as golf, tennis, volleyball or swimming at the local beach, pool or river.

- Make it fun. Be creative and explore your new surroundings by hiring some bikes or canoes, go bushwalking or have an active picnic with a kite frisbee.

- Pack some exercise equipment that is light and easy to transport, such as a skipping rope or rubber resistance strap.

Day 352 tip – Motivation and mindset

Take advantage of our slimming summers

Any time of year is a good time to be active; however, summer is the
ideal season for weight loss. In one study, people decreased body fat
during summer and autumn and increased body fat through winter and
spring. Bone and muscle mass increased after the summer/autumn period
and significantly decreased in the winter/spring period. The results are
noteworthy because the gains and losses did not balance each other out,
and by the end of the year there was a net loss of muscle in the legs and a
net gain of fat around the abdomen.

Living it

Step things up in summer by using the extra daylight hours and pleasant
weather to get outdoors and try a wider variety of activities. The warmer
temperatures also mix well with fresh foods, seafood, salads, fruits and
refreshing cool drinks of water. Don't be tempted to go on a crazy crash
diet just to get into your swimsuit. It will only make things worse in the long
run.

Day 353 tip – Good food

Sip on a smoothie (conditions apply)

Smoothies are a tasty and healthy breakfast or snack that you can mix up
in minutes. The milk or soy drink gives you protein, while the fruit gives you
sweetness, nutrients and fibre. You can also add extra fibre in the form
of grain products like psyllium husks or quick cook oats to make you feel
fuller for longer. Just soak them in the milk for a few minutes to soften them
before blending. Be aware that full-fat dairy products or a large serving size
would cancel out all the weight reducing benefits of a smoothie.

Living it

Combine your favourite ingredients and fruits to make your own smoothie.

Instead of …	Go for …
Full-fat milk, full-cream milk powder, large portions, full-fat ice-cream and full-fat yoghurt	Fresh fruit, frozen fruit, skim milk, low-fat soy milk, ice, low-fat yoghurt, skim milk powder, low-fat ice-cream, whey powder, quick cook oats, oatmeal, wheat germ, psyllium husks, nutmeg, cinnamon

Day 354 tip – Move more

Don't use sweat as a guide to a good workout

When you exercise, your body produces heat. If you have excess body fat, that heat gets insulated and you sweat even more. Sweat is produced by your skin so it evaporates and cools the blood flowing close to the surface. The amount of sweat you produce will also depend on your age, fitness level, genetics, hydration level and temperature.

Living it

Because of all the variables, sweat is not a reliable indicator of fat burning. There is no doubt that working out of a higher intensity will burn more kilojoules and make you sweat more, but the same workout on a colder day is just as beneficial, even if you sweat less. Finally, don't be embarrassed to sweat during physical activity. By generating heat and sweating, you are burning off kilojoules and you are taking action.

Day 355 tip – Motivation and mindset

Give the gift of health (you can also ask for it yourself)

Looking for some birthday or Christmas gift ideas? Why not give the gift of good health and wellness. Everyone loves to get goodies, so why not do your family and friends a favour? Try to select presents that can add year round quality of life to those you care about. Avoid things like chocolates or shortbread biscuits that are clogged with fat. They'll probably get enough of that junk from other people.

Living it

Some suggestions include health and recipe books, a pedometer, heart rate monitor, kites, frisbees, a gift certificate at a sports store or enrolling someone in a cooking class. You could also buy a 3-month membership at the local gym or a block of personal training session. Don't forget to have these kinds of gift ideas in mind when your friends and family ask what you want.

Day 356 tip – Good food

Don't always assume that a salad is healthy

What's the better choice – a hamburger or a salad? Well, the answer might surprise you. Just because it's a salad doesn't necessarily mean it's a good choice for weight loss. Many a fatty item has been bundled up under the guise of a 'salad'. For example, the chicken caesar salad at McDonald's contains nearly as much fat (22.8g) as a Big Mac (25.1g). Both are incredibly high in kilojoules and artery-clogging saturated fats and trans fats, and should be left to the very odd occasion. To give McDonald's credit, their garden mixed salad with French dressing only has 2.8 grams of fat, and is a significantly better option if your goal is to lose weight and body fat. Try to avoid creamy salads made from potato, pasta or tuna, or anything mixed with mayonnaise, cheese or sour cream. Just a few tablespoons of the wrong dressing, plus a little cheese and presto, you've converted an otherwise healthy plate of salad vegetables into a high-kilojoule, fat-storing junk food.

Living it

Look for salads with lots of vegetables, lean meats if desired, and toppings such as chickpeas, pinto beans and black beans. Add a small portion of avocado or sprinkle a few nuts and seeds on top for added flavour and some healthy fats. For the dressing, use a little bit of olive oil mixed with great options like balsamic vinegar, apple cider vinegar or lemon juice.

Day 357 tip – Move more

Take care when exercising in the heat

While spending time outdoors is a great way to add variety and enjoyment to your exercise routine, it's also a place where dehydration and heat-induced illness can occur.

Living it

Consider the following tips before starting your warm weather workout to maximise kilojoule burning and speed your recovery.

- **The right time** – Try to plan your exercise or activities during the cooler and less humid parts of the day, such as early morning or early evening. If you have to exercise in the middle of the day, follow the normal skin care rules of sunscreen, hat, sunglasses and a shirt.

- **Fluid replacement** – Make sure you drink before, during and after exercise in the heat. Don't wait till you're thirsty, as you may already be partially dehydrated. Little sips of cool water are best, while sports drinks are helpful if your activity lasts longer than 60 minutes.

- **Have a break** – Take a rest if you have been active for over an hour. You may even want to perform shorter bouts of exercise in the heat, or try a water-based activity if it's too hot.

- **Know the signs of dehydration** – Early signs of dehydration include thirst, light-headedness, tiredness, grogginess, nausea and a cold, clammy feeling. If these warning signs are ignored, more serious symptoms may develop, including heat cramps, heat exhaustion and heat stroke.

Day 358 tip – Motivation and mindset

Have a solution for your resolution

Like them or hate them, New Year's resolutions are a part of life during early January. Losing weight is the number one New Year's resolution, but most people give up within the first 2 months.

Living it

The New Year is the perfect time to start afresh and cleanse yourself of any past indulgences or bad habits. Following are some strategies that will help make your resolutions successful.

- Start today and make things happen. Be a shining example of the difference between intention and action.

- Make a commitment, not a wish. Let others know what you are trying to achieve so they can keep you accountable.

- Keep it simple by only making one or two changes at a time. By taking a long-term approach, you are much more likely to succeed.

- Have mini goals (daily or weekly) that break down your long-term goal into small, achievable steps.

- Be positive about making changes. If you have failed before, try a different strategy.

- Have a way to measure your success.

Day 359 tip – Good food

Eat well on your holidays

Holidays can be a challenging time if you are trying to eat well and look after your health.

Living it

Use the following strategies to enjoy your holiday without sacrificing your weight-loss goals.

- Look for self-contained accommodation with cooking facilities so you can prepare some of your own meals instead of having to eat out every night.

- Do your waist and your wallet a favour and leave the mini-bar treats for the next guests.

- Start the day well with a good breakfast, choosing cereals, skim milk, fruit and low-fat yoghurt instead of bacon and eggs.

- Drink plenty of water. It helps to ward off hunger, reduces your kilojoule intake and keeps you well hydrated.

- Keep your portion sizes down by eating slowly, and stop eating when you begin to feel full.

- If you drink alcohol, balance it out by eating less or eating healthier at other times of the day.

- If you must have fast food, choose from some of the healthier menu items available and keep your portions down.

Day 360 tip – Move more

Work out in water

Performing exercise in water is a great way to add variety and beat the heat, and you can exercise with a lower risk of injury. Exercise in water is ideal for people who are very overweight, pregnant, just starting an exercise program, arthritic, or those with knee or back problems. Plus, it adds cross-training variety to your exercise routine and is a refreshing way to exercise. While swimming isn't ideal for burning fat, there are other water-based activities that can help get you into shape.

Living it

Below are four water-based activities that could be a refreshing addition to your exercise routine.

- **Shallow-water walking** – Walk in water that's about ankle to knee deep while bringing your knees up high and swinging your arms to propel you. The resistance of the water builds up, helping to burn extra kilojoules.

- **Deep-water running** – Perform a free running action while wearing a buoyancy vest to prevent your feet from touching the bottom.

- **Kickboarding** – A great workout for your legs and buttocks, just hold the kickboard out with your arms straight, and pump those legs to your heart's content.

- **Aquarobics** – These classes are a great workout, and the faster you push or pull in the water, the greater the resistance will be. Check with the pools in your area to see if any classes are available.

Day 361 tip – Motivation and mindset
Don't let it all go during festive occasions like Christmas
There's no doubt that festive occasions are a challenging time if you are trying to reduce body fat. They usually revolve around large meals, large portions and lashings of alcohol to wash it all down. They can even seem to last for weeks, like Christmas and New Year's celebrations.

Living it
There are some steps you can take to make sure you enjoy yourself and still stay on track.

- **Have some quality time away from food** – One or two indulgent days is okay, but try to focus a little more on your friends and family and a little less on the food and drink. Spend some quality time together away from food. This could include a few hours at the beach, bushwalking, or having an active picnic. You could even try a sports day, such as cricket, volleyball or soccer.
- **Eat till your satisfied, not stuffed** – Ask yourself how full you feel, and if you really need that second helping. Eat slowly to keep your portion size down and stop eating when you begin to feel full. Don't continue to eat just to please others.
- **Earn your alcohol** – Alcohol is extremely high in kilojoules. If you drink more, balance it out with a little extra exercise, more water, or adjust your diet by eating less or eating more healthily.
- **Aim for maintenance** – Take a different mental approach at these times by focusing on maintaining instead of losing. You can still indulge a little while trying to minimise the damage.
- **Get straight back on the wagon** – Letting yourself go during the odd special occasions is one thing, but don't fall back into your old habits. Get back into your new healthy lifestyle habits as soon as possible.
- **Have fun** – Festive times are to be enjoyed, including food and drink. Even if you gain a kilo or two, don't be too hard on yourself. It's what you do most of the time that matters, not what you do occasionally.

Day 362 tip – Good food
Try to de-junk, not detox
Detox kits and supplements are one of the latest health fads, but can they really help you lose weight fast? In theory, a strict program of elimination and supplementation is meant to rid your body of impurities and flush out

bowels. In reality, there is no proven scientific evidence to support specific detox diets, programs or supplement kits. Cutting out whole food groups can actually deprive your body of essential nutrients, while severe kilojoule restriction can deplete muscle and slow down your metabolic rate (although it will look good on the scales for a few weeks). Any program that encourages you to eat less junk food, cut out cigarettes, reduce your alcohol intake, eat more vegetables and drink more water will benefit your health. These changes will help you lose weight and make you feel better, but there's nothing magical about the detox diet itself. It's actually the lifestyle changes that benefit your health. You can boost your body's natural functioning by adopting good habits every day, rather than purchasing a 2-week kit.

Living it

Look for ways to bring your diet back to basics without taking supplements or eliminating whole food groups. Cut back on saturated fats and excess kilojoules, especially from takeaway meals, alcohol, sugar and processed foods.

Day 363 tip – Move more

Use the beach – the most versatile gym in the world

Whether you are lucky enough to live near the ocean or just visiting on holidays, there's so much you can do at the beach. Some activities may require a little extra gear, while others you can do without any equipment, and many you can do all year round. After you've burnt off all those kilojoules, you can cool off with a dip in the water, and leave feeling strong, well and refreshed.

Living it

Following is a list of the types of activities you can combine or do on their own, making the beach a workout wonderland:

- walking and running on the sand (soft and hard)
- walking and running in ankle- to knee-deep water
- swimming laps in the ocean pool
- swimming in the open water
- bodysurfing
- paddling on a wave ski
- surfing
- body boarding
- sprinting on the sand and up sand dunes
- beach volleyball

- body weight circuits – combining cardio with exercises like push-ups and lunges
- surfboat rowing.

Day 364 tip – Motivation and mindset

Focus on how far you've come, and congratulate yourself on a journey well started

We have covered so much together, and I hope you have learnt a lot. But the journey doesn't end here. I hope you continue to learn, continue to eat well, continue to achieve personal best results with your exercise, continue to stay motivated, and continue to find joy in the process of healthy living.

Living it

My hope is that you have already been 'living it'. Look back on what tips you have adopted since the start of *Lighten Up*, and focus on the positive steps you have made. You could also look back over some of the tips that didn't hit the mark with you at the time because you may be in a different mindset now and feel better prepared to take them on board. Please email me with any questions, concerns, success stories or feedback you have, and while you're at it, subscribe to my free weekly email newsletter. Just go to my website **www.andrewcate.com**. I look forward to hearing from you.

Day 365 tip – Good food

Enjoy a healthy BBQ (conditions apply)

A weekend BBQ with family and friends is a fantastic part of our way of life, but don't let it become a kilojoule blow out.

Living it

You can get pretty creative with healthy foods on a BBQ. Make some tasty treats for your guests, or take along your own when visiting others. Healthy food choices can taste just as good as traditional, and often less healthy, alternatives – as you can see below.

Instead of ...	Go for ...
Potato crisps	Unbuttered popcorn, rice crackers and salsa
Sausages	Lean beef
Chicken with skin	Marinated skinless chicken breast
Large portions	Small meat portions, and extra grilled vegetables
Creamy salads	Garden salads with balsamic vinegar and a little oil

'I lost 25kg over 12 months following Andrew's advice. I went from being sedentary to becoming a regular walker and enjoying the experience. Andrew's book kept me motivated, and really helped me shed those kilos! And furthermore, I enjoyed the experience'

Inge

'Two years ago, I was de-motivated, overweight and tired all the time. I knew I should of been exercising, but didn't have the knowledge or drive to do anything about it. After reading Andrew's book, something clicked. I got fitter, lost weight, and gained the confidence to try new things. I am now representing Australia in dragon boating. Thanks Andrew.'

Hillary

'It's been an incredible transformation. I've lost weight steadily and over my entire body so now my rings and sandals are also loose – not just my clothes. I've even wondered at times if I might have had a mystery illness and the weight loss was a coincidence – it's been so complete and fast. But I have regular health checks and everything is A-OK. I've never felt better'.

Lyndal

'I have recently purchased your book, and wanted to let you know that I found it fantastic! I have found your book to be very motivating, it has given me all the information and facts that I need, without all the mumbo-jumbo. It's concise, straight-forward approach is very helpful, and it has excellent suggestions and tips to help me (and others) succeed. I will be recommending your book to others.'

Melanie

'Just want to say I found your book to be a treasure trove of gems for losing weight. Your book is just what I needed to get out of the stalemate I was in. Thank you once again for the Motivation that I needed to start afresh.'

Gary

Thank you for your book. It's easy to read, easy to follow and actually made me feel like I could do something about my state.'

Janet